Larry — May 1997

For all of your contributions to the field of Oculomotor control.

Ken C.

ACCOMMODATION, NEARWORK AND MYOPIA

Editha Ong, O.D., Ph.D.

Kenneth J. Ciuffreda, O.D., Ph.D.

Optometric Extension Program

Printed in the United States of America

Published by Optometric Extension Program Foundation, Inc.
1921 East Carnegie Ave., 3-L
Santa Ana, CA 92705-5510

Library of Congress Cataloging in Publication data
Ong, Editha.
Accommodation, nearwork and myopia / Editha Ong, Kenneth J. Ciuffreda.
p. cm.
Includes bibliographical references.
ISBN 0-943599-88-1 (alk. paper)
1. Myopia—Etiology. 2. Eye—Accommodation and refraction. I. Ciuffreda, Kenneth J., 1947- . II. Title.
[DNLM: 1. Myopia—etiology. 2. Accommodation, Ocular. WW 320 058a 1997]
RE938.054 1997
617.7'55—dc21
DNLM/DLC
for Library of Congress 96-51078
CIP

DEDICATIONS

To our families.

To Mom and Dad, for your vision.

To Chris and Nikki, for your inspiration.
E.O.

To my mother for always being there.
K.J.C.

"...............refractive state is largely programmed on a genetic basis, but an abnormal visual experience can disrupt the process of postnatal growth and induce axial myopia."

Raviola and Wiesel

"Heredity establishes the potentialities, but environment may decide the actualities."

Duke-Elder

"If refractive errors can be produced, it should be possible to prevent their occurrence or even cure them."

Grosvenor and Flom

TABLE OF CONTENTS

FOREWORD

There is perhaps no other topic that fascinates optometrists more than myopia. And, of equal fascination, at least to those who subscribe to a function-behavioral basis for visual problems, is the determination of its etiology. While genetic, nutritional, and psychological causes have been proposed and endured, the question of whether the complex of near work and accommodation is a, if not *the,* major etiological component for myopia has increasingly gained stature. However, there are strong adherents to the pro and con sides of this question; indeed, discussions often become arguments, and friendships have been modified because of differing opinions. It is certainly not a trite question, because the side one takes determines the treatment options offered to patients.

In this monograph, Drs. Ong and Ciuffreda offer us the most complete and current review of the relationship between near work and accommodation to the onset and continuance of myopia. To their credit, they have accomplished this in a very readable and clinically-relevant manner. The closed -minded reader will probably not be receptive when his or her beliefs are challenged on the basis of sound research; on the other hand, the open-minded reader will perhaps change some of his or her convictions, come away intellectually richer, and provide more enlightened patient care.

It is particularly fitting that this monograph is published by the Optometric Extension Program (OEP). For, while others had raised the issue previously, it was the late Dr. A. M. Skeffington, a founder of OEP, who most succinctly made the case that the "socially compulsive" yet "biologically unacceptable" nearpoint tasks that are unique to societies based in the written word were responsible for the development of visual problems. He certainly viewed the onset and continuance of certain myopias in this regard.[1] Ong and Ciuffreda essentially investigate Skeffington's hypothesis with the benefit of research, knowledge and technology that was not available during his lifetime in an open, yet scholarly manner. I have no doubt that Dr. Skeffington would have been the most avid reader of this monograph.

Irwin B. Suchoff, O.D., D.O.S.
Distinguished Service Professor
State University of New York
State College of Optometry
New York City

References

1. Skeffington AM. Nearpoint optometry. Santa Ana, Calif: Optom Exten Prog; 1950 (6):1.

PREFACE

Yet another work on the topic of accommodation, nearwork and myopia? That certainly is a reasonable question to ask given the hundreds of published papers, abstracts and proceedings, monographs and books, theses, etc., already available in this area. Our book's "raison d'etre" is perhaps best exemplified by the title of the last chapter, "Myopia: Past, Present and Future." To us, there appeared to be much unclear thinking and confusion about the interpretation of past endeavors, little summary of the current state of affairs, and some reluctance to provide guidance and speculation as to possible future directions.

Thus, the birth of our monograph. Chapter 1 provides an overview of accommodation, the process and ramifications of which are central to the book's theme. In Chapter 2, the reader is given a detailed and up-to-date critical account of accommodation in myopia, with comparison of these findings to the other refractive groups. Thus, one learns just how well (or badly) the myope accommodates. And, in Chapter 3, the effect of nearwork on both the onset and development of permanent myopia in various targeted populations is considered, as this link is critical to our arguments. Chapter 4 reviews, summarizes, and offers new insights and speculations regarding the role of transient, nearwork-induced myopia in the overall picture of myopigenesis. In Chapter 5, the biomechanics of accommodation and convergence are detailed and critically reviewed with respect to their potential role in myopia, with this information having served for many years as a source of considerable confusion and misperception. Chapter 6 begins to develop the unique idea that perhaps it is not the mechanical process of accommodation per se but rather the resultant retinal defocus which may serve as the primary myopigenic factor. Finally, in Chapter 7, an attempt has been made to provide brief summary accounts of the important topical issues in the area and to suggest future new and perhaps controversial ways to approach the important refractive condition of myopia.

Editha Ong, O.D., Ph.D.
Kenneth J. Ciuffreda, O.D., Ph.D.
New York City
October 1996

ACKNOWLEDGEMENTS

We thank the New York Academy of Optometry, the Optometric Extension Program Foundation, the College of Optometrists in Vision Development, and the Schnurmacher Institute for Vision Research at the SUNY/State College of Optometry for their financial support to E. O. as a post-doctoral fellow with K.J.C.

We thank Drs. W. Bleything, K. Citek and I.B. Suchoff for reading the entire manuscript, and Dr. N.A. McBrien for reviewing Chapter 5.

ABOUT THE AUTHORS

Editha Ong received her O.D. degree from Centro Escolar University, Manila, and her M.S. and Ph.D. degrees in vision science from SUNY/State College of Optometry in New York City under the direction of Dr. Kenneth J. Ciuffreda. During her post-doctoral fellowship, this monograph was completed. Her research areas include accommodation and myopia.

Kenneth J. Ciuffreda received his B.A. in biology from Seton Hall University, his O.D. degree from the Massachusetts College of Optometry and his Ph.D. degree in physiological optics from the University of California, Berkeley, in the School of Optometry. He has been a faculty member at SUNY/State College of Optometry in New York City since 1979, where he is presently Chairman, Department of Vision Sciences and Distinguished Teaching Professor. He is also an Associate Member of the Graduate Faculty in Biomedical Engineering at Rutgers University in New Jersey. His research areas include eye movements, accommodation, myopia, amblyopia, and bioengineering applications to clinical optometry. Dr. Ciuffreda has over 170 publications, with this being his fifth book.

CHAPTER 1
OVERVIEW OF ACCOMMODATION

Accommodation refers to the process whereby a minimal diameter retinal blur circle is obtained by appropriate alteration in the dioptric power of the crystalline lens (See Ciuffreda 1991, in press, for detailed reviews) (Figure 1-1), thereby maximizing retinal image contrast (Heath 1956b). Hence, the accommodative system is primarily driven and controlled by the retinal blur aspect of a visual stimulus. Nevertheless, it also has numerous other visual and non-visual inputs that can influence the response (Ciuffreda 1991, in press). The overall response is generally considered to be a non-linearly-additive aggregate of four components classified according to their stimulus characteristics (Heath 1956b). These include blur or "reflex" accommodation, proximal accommodation, vergence accommodation, and tonic accommodation. This classification is analogous to that proposed by Maddox (1893) for vergence. See Figure 1-2.

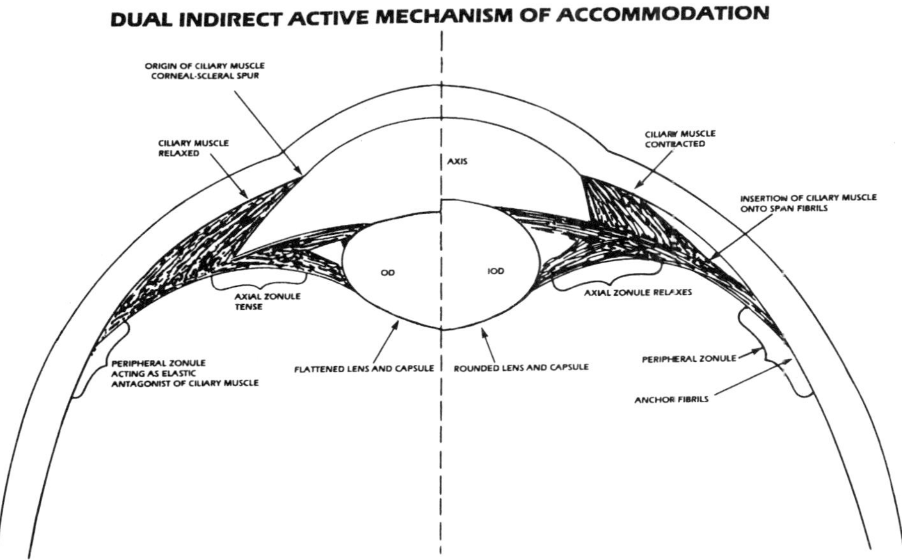

Figure 1-1 : The eye in sagittal section. Shows important accommodative structures in the anterior third of the eye for both decreased (left) and increased (right) accommodation (Reprinted with permission, Stark 1988).

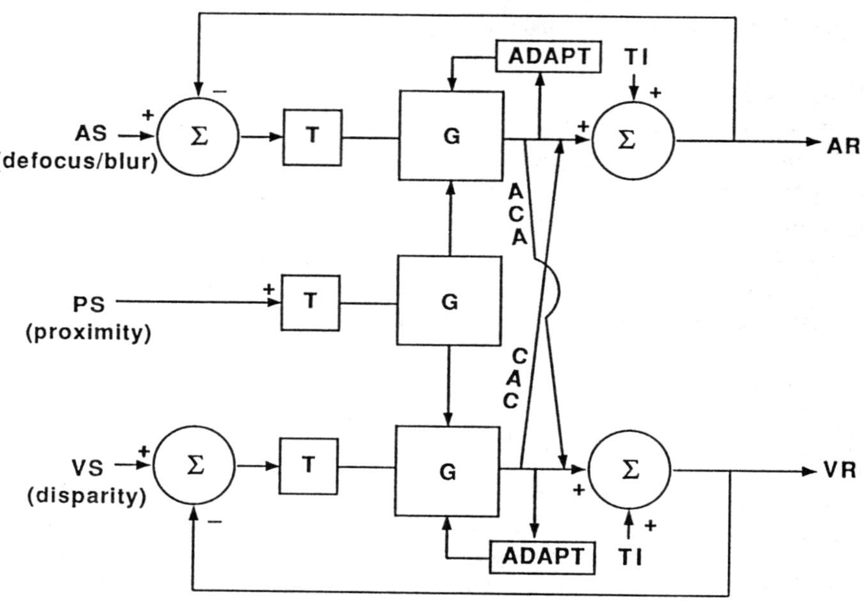

Figure 1-2 : Steady-state model of the accommodative and vergence systems. Symbols: AS= accommodative stimulus, VS= disparity stimulus, PS= proximal stimulus. AR = accommodative response, VR = vergence response, Σ= summing junction for various inputs, T= threshold detector, G= system gain, ADAPT= adaptive component, ACA= accommodative convergence to accommodation (crosslink gain), CAC= convergence accommodation to convergence (crosslink gain), and TI= tonic input (Reprinted with permission, Ciuffreda 1992).

COMPONENTS OF ACCOMMODATION (Heath 1956b, Ciuffreda 1991, in press)

1) Blur or "reflex" accommodation

Blur was regarded by Heath (1956b) as the primary drive to accommodation. Reflex accommodation refers to the automatic adjustment of the refractive state of the eye in response to blur, which probably reflects changes in the retinal-image contrast gradient, to attain and maintain maximal retinal-image contrast and clarity. Reflex accommodation is responsive to smaller amounts of blur, up to approximately 2D or so (Fincham 1951). It is constrained optically by the ocular depth-of-focus.

2) Proximal accommodation

This refers to accommodation elicited by knowledge of the apparent or perceived nearness of an object. It can also be evoked to some extent by mental imagery, e.g., by merely "thinking near." It is typically measured under special blur-free or "open-loop" conditions in which a subject is made aware of the proximity of the target and nearby surrounds. Instrument myopia is a manifestation of proximal accommodation.

3) Vergence accommodation

Due to the neural link from disparity (or fusional) vergence to the accommodative system (Ciuffreda and Kenyon 1983), all vergence movements are accompanied by a corresponding accommodative change, the magnitude of which is dependent upon the individual's convergence accommodation-to-convergence, or CA/C ratio. Hence, vergence accommodation refers to the amount of accommodation evoked by the act of vergence, with the latter being stimulated by retinal disparity.

4) Tonic accommodation

In the absence of the aforementioned three components, for example in a large and totally darkened room, the accommodative system reverts to its tonic accommodative state (Rosenfield et al. 1993). This is also referred to as dark focus, the resting state of accommodation, or abias. It probably reflects baseline midbrain neural activity (Fisher et al 1987). Thus, tonic accommodation refers to the refractive state of the eye when visual feedback has been rendered ineffective, e.g., when the accommodative and vergence systems are rendered open-loop with the use of pinholes and occlusion, respectively, to remove both blur and disparity, and when all proximal, cognitive, and other such influences are either absent or minimal. Tonic accommodation is typically assessed in total darkness, under contrastless "ganzfeld" conditions, or with the use of a pinhole under otherwise normal monocular viewing conditions. Tonic accommodation has been reported to have a mean value of approximately 1.50D (Leibowitz and Owens 1978), although recent data using more optimal open-field instrumentation reveals a lower average value of 0.5 to 1D in young adults (Rosenfield et al. 1993). Nocturnal myopia and space myopia may be regarded as manifestations of tonic accommodation.

STATIC ASPECTS OF ACCOMMODATION

Accommodative Stimulus/Response Function

The accommodative stimulus/response function provides a measure of steady-state accommodation over a range of dioptric inputs (Figure 1-3) (Ciuffreda and Kenyon 1983; Ciuffreda 1991, in press). This can be generated by altering optical vergence of the target either by varying target distance in physical space, target position within a Badal optical system or

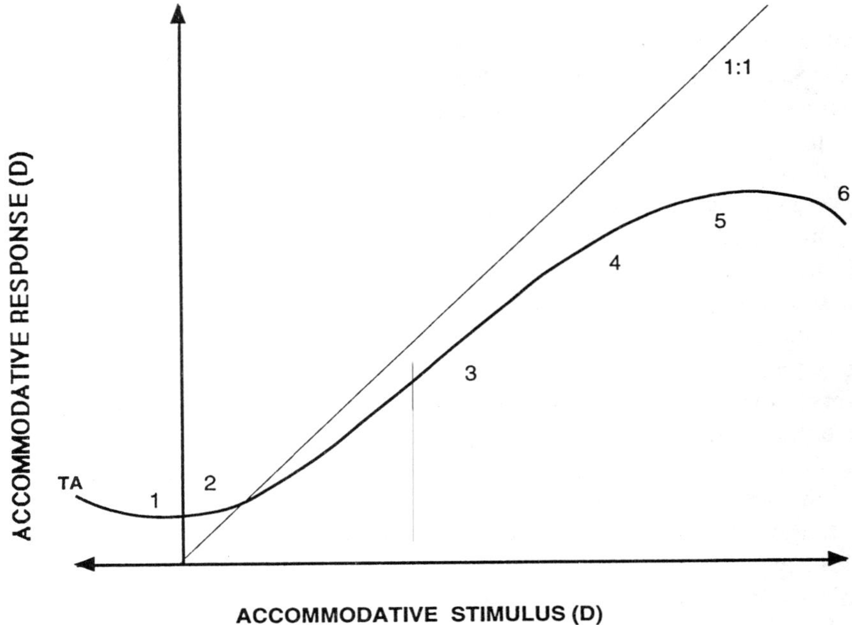

Figure 1-3 : Accommodative stimulus/response curve. Typically, a target is moved within a Badal optical system from beyond optical infinity to a value closer than the near point of accommodation, and the steady-state accommodative response at a variety of stimulus levels is ascertained. TA=tonic accommodative level, and 1:1=equidioptric stimulus/response line.

with spherical lenses placed in front of the eyes. A typical response profile exhibits: (a) a depth-of-focus-related/hyperfocal refraction-biased lead for farther stimulus distances (i.e., beyond 2 meters or so), (b) a lag at closer stimulus distances (i.e., nearer than 1 meter or so), with a typical gain (i.e., the accommodative stimulus divided by the accommodative response) in the mid-linear region of approximately 0.7 to 0.9 (Ciuffreda et al. 1984, Ong et al. 1993), and (c) an accommodative error at near that is proportional to the accommodative stimulus (e.g., a proportional neural controller, Toates 1972), so that increasing lags are found for progressively higher stimulus levels. More specifically, the accommodative stimulus/response function is generally divided into the following six regions (Figure 1-3):

1) Hyperopic defocus region:

If the dioptric stimulus is progressively positioned *beyond* optical infinity (only possible in optical systems), the accommodative response gradually shifts (relative to the response at optical infinity) slightly higher towards the tonic accommodative level. This increased overaccommodation is elicited due to inability of the accommodative system to achieve clarity of the target i.e., one cannot accommodate beyond optical infinity if fully corrected, with the resultant non-compensatible retinal defocus driving the system towards its "default" tonic level.

2) Initial non-linear zone:
This is typically characterized by a lead of accommodation. It encompasses stimulus levels ranging from 0 to approximately 1.5D. This response region is primarily influenced by tonic accommodation and the depth-of-focus (Hung and Semmlow 1980).

3) Linear manifest zone:
Over this region, a change in accommodative stimulus produces a corresponding proportional change in accommodative response, and a depth-of-focus-based "lazy" lag of accommodation is typically evident. This is the primary region over which steady-state accommodation at near is assessed both experimentally and clinically.

4) "Soft" saturation zone:
This non-linear region is characterized by increasingly smaller changes in accommodative response for progressively greater increases in the accommodative stimulus. Thus, the lag of accommodation, and hence its static or steady-state error, progressively increases with further increases in accommodative stimulus level.

5) "Hard" saturation zone:
This region is non-linear as well. Further changes in the accommodative stimulus are no longer capable of eliciting any change in accommodative response. The initial portion of this zone represents the clinical amplitude of accommodation.

6) Myopic defocus region:
This is encountered when the accommodative stimulus exceeds the individual's amplitude of accommodation by approximately 1 to 2D, producing increased amounts of underaccommodation and consequent retinal-image defocus. Beyond this point, the accommodative response becomes progressively smaller and gradually shifts toward the tonic accommodative level.

DYNAMIC ASPECTS OF ACCOMMODATION

Step Input

The accommodative system responds with a mean latency of 360 and 380 ms for a far-to-near and a near-to-far rapid step change in stimulus, respectively (Campbell and Westheimer 1960). Such changes in the accommodative stimulus occur, for example, when looking from far-to-near or with interposition of a minus lens over the eye. Furthermore, it has been shown that the mean latency was markedly reduced and even negative for predictable step inputs (Phillips et al. 1972), as one might expect. The mean lens movement times were 640 ms for far-to-near accommodation and 560 ms for near-to-far randomized or non-predictable shifts in focus. Therefore, the total time interval (i.e., latency plus lens movement time) between the onset of a stimulus and the attainment of a new level of steady-state accommodation was approximately one second for single movement responses (Campbell and Westheimer 1960). The accommodative response profile is characterized by a decreasing exponential function, with a time constant (i.e., the time to attain 63% of its intended movement or response change) of approximately 200 to 250 ms (Campbell and Westheimer 1960), although response range non-linearities were evident for time constants but not for latencies (Shirachi et al. 1978). For example, increasing accommodation (far-to-near) was faster when initiated at far (255 ms) than at near (440 ms). This asymmetry was also evident but reversed for decreasing accommodation (near-to-far). Accommodation was now faster at near (320 ms) relative to far (440 ms). These were attributed to the mechanical constraints of the peripheral accommodative apparatus, i.e., the lens and ciliary muscle. Response peak velocity increased with a ratio of 4 or 5 to 1 as a function of response amplitude (Schnider et al. 1984). Thus, maximum velocity for a 2D response was 10D/sec (Campbell and Westheimer 1960). Accommodative amplitude and velocity also exhibited diurnal variations (Randle and Murphy 1974). And, lastly, the dynamic response characteristics for both reflex and voluntary accommodation were found to be the same (Campbell and Westheimer 1960, Randle and Murphy 1974, Ciuffreda and Kruger 1988), suggesting similar lower-level control aspects despite dissimilar higher-level initiation (Ciuffreda and Kruger 1988).

Sinusoidal and Ramp Inputs

Responses to sinusoidally-varying accommodative inputs (i.e., target velocity is maximal at midrange and zero at either end) showed frequency-related changes (Campbell and Westheimer 1960). The response amplitude (i.e., gain) decreased, and the phase lag (i.e., lag of the response behind the target movement) increased, with such a target having a fixed amplitude but increasingly higher temporal frequencies (Campbell and Westheimer 1960).

The gain and phase lag were found to increase and decrease, respectively, when such tracking was repeated over a period of time, suggesting a moderate practice effect (Randle and Murphy 1974). For ramp or constant-velocity stimuli, the accommodative system responded smoothly to slow ramp velocities, but became more discrete and step-like with increasing velocities (Hung and Ciuffreda 1988). Furthermore, Hung and Ciuffreda (1988) suggested that the accommodative system exhibited dual-mode behavior, i.e., a pre-programmed mode characterizing the initial 200 msec or so rapid response component reflecting the "fast" system, and a continuous visual feedback monitoring mode characterizing the latter 500 msec or so of the response reflecting the "slow" system.

Pulse Input

Data on accommodation in response to rapid pulse inputs of brief durations (i.e., less than the accommodative system latency, or reaction time) reflected its apparent continuous input sampling nature for such target changes (but see the above dual-mode argument). That is, information regarding the state of focus was continually being obtained, even while an accommodative movement was in progress (Campbell and Westheimer 1960). Therefore, accommodation could be modified, at least during some portions of the actual motor response.

Microfluctuations

The accommodative response constantly exhibits oscillations of a small magnitude (± 0.1D or so) (Charman and Heron 1988). These oscillations are generally more pronounced at both the slower (0.01 to 0.5 Hz) and faster (1.5 to 2 Hz) range than elsewhere over the 5 Hz total bandwidth of response (Campbell et al. 1959). The fluctuations were maximal at intermediate and near distances, and progressively decreased for either very close or very far distances (Miege and Denieul 1988), presumably due to biomechanical limitations of the zonules (Ciuffreda 1991). Microfluctuations were suggested to be central in origin due to their consensuality (Campbell 1960). The role of the 2 Hz component was originally suggested to provide directional cues to accommodation (Campbell et al. 1959, Kotulak and Schor 1986), but more recent evidence suggested it was due to biological noise related to cardiac pulse rate (Winn et al. 1990). However, the lower frequency oscillations probably assist in steady-state accommodative accuracy (Charman and Heron 1988).

ANATOMICAL ASPECTS OF ACCOMMODATION

Crystalline Lens/Lens Capsule

Thomas Young (1801) was the first to identify correctly the role of the crystalline lens during the process of accommodation. The lens is a transparent, elastic, and avascular structure enclosed within an elastic capsule (Alpern 1969). Lens growth occurs throughout life. New fibers are produced at the equator, and then grow and elongate towards the anterior and posterior surfaces (Weale 1982). Each successive layer of lens fibers has a different index of refraction, with the lens core having the greatest index (Gullstrand 1908). The lens capsule which envelopes the lens also grows throughout life due to the division of epithelial cells at the equator (Alpern 1969). Its thickness varies, with the posterior pole being the thinnest and the zone 2-3mm from the anterior pole being the thickest. During increased accommodation, several lens changes occur, primarily at its anterior surface (Fincham 1937, Alpern 1969, Wyatt 1988, Ciuffreda 1991, in press). As the ciliary muscle contracts and shifts inward and anteriorly, two events occur: (1) the elastic choroid is stretched with its edge shifted anteriorly, and (2) zonular tension is reduced. The latter allows the lens capsule to exert its tension on the lens substance. The elastic properties of the lens causes slight protrusion in the central anterior surface in the area where the lens capsule is thinnest. This results in the anterior pole bulging forward during increased accommodation, giving rise to a hyperbolic profile. During maximal accommodation in a young person, the central anterior radius of curvature of the lens becomes reduced from 12 to 5 mm, while the posterior radius of curvature undergoes relatively minor changes from approximately 5.5 to 5 mm (Fincham 1937). The anterior lens pole advances forward by 0.3 mm, while the posterior lens pole probably moves back by less than half that amount (Fincham 1937). Lastly, the lens increases its central thickness by approximately 0.5 mm, while its equatorial diameter decreases by about 0.4 mm (Fincham 1937). The reverse occurs with decreasing accommodation. However, it should be noted that now the choroid is primarily responsible for displacing the ciliary muscle back to its original position via its elastic spring action (Wyatt 1988).

Ciliary Muscle

The ciliary muscle consists of a ring of smooth muscle adjacent to the inner surface of the anterior sclera (Moses 1987). Since it comprises the anterior portion of the uveal tract, the ciliary muscle is effectively continuous with the choroid (Alpern 1969). The muscle fibers originate at the corneo-scleral spur and insert at the span fibrils of the Zonules of Zinn at Bruch's membrane (Rohen 1979, Stark 1988). Contraction of the ciliary muscle results in axipetal displacement (i.e., forward and inward) of the zonular attachment, with a forward pulling of the choroid (Moses 1987). Contraction pulls on the span fibrils, which in turn produces increased tension in the peripheral portion of the zonules (Stark 1988). This frees the axial portion of the zonules and allows the lens to assume a rounder shape (Figure 1-1). The ciliary muscle fibers traditionally have been categorized according to the orientation of their fiber length (Salzmann 1912). These include: (1) the longitudinal fibers, also known as meridional or Brueck's muscle, which run antero-posteriorly, (2) the circular fibers (sphincter or Mueller's muscle), which are the innermost fibers, run circumferentially around the globe, and (3) the third muscle group, the radial fibers, connect the other two groups of muscles. These three groups appear as a tangled meshwork, however, and in reality constitute a single muscle of unitary function.

Zonulus of Zinn

The suspensory ligament of the lens, otherwise known as the Zonulus of Zinn, consists of a series of delicate acellular fibrils (Alpern 1969). They run longitudinally from the pars plana of the ciliary body and anastomose with one other (Rohen 1979). At the level of the pars plicata, interlacing zonular plexuses are formed and are attached to the lateral walls of the ciliary processes (Rohen 1979). Further anteriorly, the zonular plexusus appears to proceed at an angle and finally split into the "zonular fork" (Rohen 1979), which attaches to the zonular lamellae of the lens capsule (Alpern 1969, Rohen 1979). The zonular attachment to the lens capsule was found to be segregated into three groups. The two more prominent ones composing the "zonular fork" attached to the anterior and posterior lens capsule, while the less dense one attached to the equator (Rohen 1979, Moses 1987). Some of the zonules also run meridionally within the ciliary body itself (Moses 1987), while others run posteriorly to the vitreous and ora serrata (McCulloch 1954, Moses 1987).

NEUROPHYSIOLOGY OF ACCOMMODATION

The afferent pathway commences with the stimulation of cones by a defocussed retinal image (Campbell 1954, Heath 1956a). The blur signals generated by the cones pass through the magnocellular layer of the lateral geniculate body (Kaplan and Shapley 1982) and are then transmitted to cortical area 17 (Dean 1981). The signal is then passed on to the parieto-temporal areas for further processing (Jampel 1959, Harrison 1987, Ohtsuka et al. 1988). The neural signal is transformed into a motor command at the midbrain-oculomotor nucleus complex/Edinger-Westphal nucleus (Jaeger and Benevento 1980, Judge and Cummings 1986). The efferent pathway includes the third cranial nerve (oculomotor nerve), the ciliary ganglion, and the short ciliary nerve which ultimately innervates the ciliary muscle (Netter 1962). Contraction of the ciliary muscle results in correlated changes of the crystalline lens and related structures as described above. See Ciuffreda (1991, in press) for detailed overviews.

PHARMACOLOGY OF ACCOMMODATION

The accommodative system receives mutually-antagonistic, dual innervation from the autonomic nervous system. It is composed primarily of a parasympathetic and secondarily a sympathetic component (Gilmartin et al. 1992). The parasympathetic input is mediated by the action of acetylcholine on muscarinic receptors, whose excitation or increased stimulation results in increased accommodation, and whose inhibition or decreased stimulation results in decreased accommodation (Biggs et al. 1959, Tornqvist 1967). The parasympathetic system is characterized by a rapid temporal response that is completed in 1-2 seconds (Campbell and Westheimer 1960), and it is the primary (probably sole) innervational component involved in the rapid changes in accommodation one makes during naturalistic viewing conditions. On the other hand, the sympathetic component is mediated by the action of noradrenaline on adrenoceptors which can further be classified into the following subtypes: alpha-1, beta-1 and beta-2. Its action is antagonistic to that of the parasympathetic component, with an innervation that is characterized as inhibitory in nature thereby resulting in decreased or "negative" accommodation (Gilmartin et al. 1984, Gilmartin 1986). Sympathetic response magnitude is related to the concurrent level of background parasympathetic activity, but it is generally much smaller with a maximal effect of only 1.5D or so (Tornqvist 1967). It also exhibits a delayed temporal response occurring over a period of 10-40 seconds (Tornqvist 1967). Thus, the role of sympathetic innervation in response to our daily visual demands which are characterized by multiple and rapid changes in accommodative level is probably minimal. However, it has been suggested that sympathetic action may be more relevant to sustained near tasks (Gilmartin and Hogan 1985b), perhaps being involved in attenuating the retention of near-induced, post-task distance pseudomyopic (i.e., lenticular-based) changes (Gilmartin and Bullimore 1987), thereby reducing the magnitude and duration of any accommodative adaptation aftereffects.

Evidence for the dominant role of the parasympathetic component was clearly manifested in an in vivo pharmacological study by Biggs et al. (1959). Topical application of parasympatholytic agents such as cyclopentolate and homatropine practically obliterated all accommodation and occasionally caused recession of the far point (Biggs et al. 1959). In contrast, subconjunctival injection of non-selective sympathomimetics such as epinephrine resulted in less dramatic accommodative changes. The primary change occurred in the accommodative amplitude which exhibited a marked reduction of 2.5D, while constancy was maintained for both the far point of accommodation and the slope of the accommodative stimulus/response function (Biggs et al. 1959).

The majority of investigators believed that the sympathetic input was mediated primarily by the inhibitory beta-adrenergic receptors (Hurwitz et al. 1972a, 1972b, Van Alphen 1976, Stephens 1985), predominantly of the beta-2 subtype (Lograno and Reibaldi 1986, Wax and Molinoff 1987, Zetterstrom and Hahnenberger 1988). In vitro experiments showed that the adrenoceptor distribution of the ciliary muscle was species-dependent, and furthermore that human eyes either showed a predominance of beta receptors (Van Alphen 1976, Lograno and Reibaldi 1986) or the presence of both alpha-1 and beta-2 receptors (Zetterstrom and Hahnenberger 1988). However, in the latter study, the investigators acknowledged that inter-subject variations in adrenoceptor subtype distribution may exist. In vivo investigations using human subjects have not been any more conclusive. The use of beta-adrenergic agonists, e.g., isoproterenol, and antagonists, e.g., timolol and betaxolol, have resulted in an absence of significant shifts in accommodative amplitude (Gilmartin et al. 1984, Gilmartin and Hogan 1985a, Zetterstrom 1988), far point (Gilmartin et al. 1984, Gilmartin and Hogan 1985a, Zetterstrom 1988), and tonic accommodation (Bullimore and Gilmartin 1987, Gilmartin and Bullimore 1987, Zetterstrom 1988). However, other studies were able to demonstrate significant beta-adrenergic-induced accommodative changes. Gilmartin et al. (1984) found a mean myopic shift of 0.85D in tonic accommodation following the administration of timolol maleate, whereas Gilmartin and Hogan (1985a) found a hyperopic shift of 0.47D with isoprenaline. The discrepancy in findings between these studies may partially be attributed to the type of instrumentation used (Gilmartin and Bullimore 1987). Bullimore and Gilmartin (1987) and Gilmartin and Bullimore (1987) used infrared optometers, while Gilmartin and colleagues (1984) used a laser optometer. The use of a laser optometer, which involved a cognitive demand by the subject to discriminate the direction of speckle motion, may have initiated a transient parasympathetic response. And, the increase in parasympathetic level might provide sufficient background activity to enable the sympathetic response to become manifested (Bullimore and Gilmartin 1987). However, perhaps a better explanation is that the studies which showed no significant changes (Bullimore and Gilmartin 1987, Gilmartin and Bullimore 1987, Zetterstrom 1988) used subjects who exhibited low levels of tonic accommodation (<1D). Since tonic accommodation has been demonstrated to be primarily parasympathetically-mediated (Gilmartin and Hogan 1985a), the presence of such low tonic accommodative levels would mean that the concurrent level of parasympathetic innervation may have been insufficient to allow the effect of sympathetic input to become manifested.

Evidence in support of the relative importance of the role of the alpha-1 subtype of adrenoceptors has not proven to be any more convincing and has remained a debated issue. In vivo human experiments have been inconclusive with regard to the accommodative response, with emphasis on tonic accommodation and the near point of accommodation. Administration of alpha-1-adrenergic agents, more specifically phenylephrine, failed to produce any significant change in either tonic accommodation (Leibowitz and Owens 1975, Garner et al. 1983, Rosenfield et al. 1990) or the far point (Leibowitz and Owens 1975, Garner 1983). In contrast, Zetterstrom (1988) reported an increase in tonic accommodation of 0.9D and a far point myopic shift of 3D, both of which she attributed to the mydriatic action associated with the administration of the pharmacological agent, since the use of 2mm artificial pupils on a few selected subjects negated all effects. In addition, thymoxamine, a non-selective alpha-antagonist, failed to induce any changes in tonic accommodation (Zetterstrom 1988, Rosenfield et al. 1990).

The pharmacological effect on alpha-receptors was better illustrated at the near point. The topical instillation of alpha-adrenergic agents, such as phenylephrine, resulted in a reduced accommodative amplitude ranging from 0.50 to 3D (Biggs 1959, Garner et al. 1983, Zetterstrom 1984, 1987, 1988, Rosenfield et al. 1990). This effect was dose-dependent, with accommodation decreasing exponentially with increasing dosage of phenylephrine (Zetterstrom 1984). And, administration of a non-selective alpha-adrenergic antagonist such as thymoxamine resulted in an increased accommodative amplitude of 0.50 to 1.50D (Rosenfield et al. 1990, Zetterstrom 1987, 1988). These findings on accommodative amplitude using alpha agonists are more consistent with the view that alpha-adrenoceptors can indeed influence accommodation. The most probable reason for the effect being manifested only at the accommodative amplitude was that sympathetically-derived influences were activated maximally in the presence of a sufficiently large concurrent parasympathetic activity, as discussed earlier.

The mechanism whereby sympathetic input influences the accommodative response has been suggested by some investigators to be indirect and vascular in nature (Morgan 1946, Fleming and Hall 1959, Gilmartin et al. 1984). Since increased alpha-innervation leads to vasoconstriction, this would result in reduced volume (and mass) of the ciliary body; this would cause an outward and backward mechanically-based shift of the ciliary body, which in turn would increase zonular tension and thereby flatten the crystalline lens. Similar effects were also hypothesized when the alpha receptors were indirectly stimulated with administration of selective sympatholytics such as beta-antagonists. For example, timolol maleate blocks beta receptors, which would result in an accumulation of noradrenaline at the synapse. The excess neurotransmitter may diffuse into the ciliary body causing vasoconstriction by virtue of the alpha receptors present in the ciliary vessels. And as discussed previously, this would indirectly produce changes in the dioptric power of the crystalline lens. However, the results of some in vitro experiments (Cogan 1937, Zetterstrom and Hahnenberger 1988) have indicated otherwise. Using isolated ciliary muscle strips which were devoid of their vascular system, changes in ciliary muscle contraction were still evident with the use of adrenergic pharmacological agents. These studies therefore demonstrated that the adrenergic response of the ciliary muscle was directly induced and was not an indirect consequence of vasculature changes.

Since sympathetically-mediated temporal responses are 10 to 20 times slower than parasympathetic responses, it has been argued that sympathetic function may be primarily related to sustained near visual tasks (Gilmartin and Hogan 1985a,b). Upon completion of such a task, a rapid decay of the parasympathetic component occurs, while the considerably more prolonged decay of the sympathetic component is reflected as accommodative adaptation in the dark and as nearwork-induced transient myopia in the light with visual feedback present. Attenuation of the sympathetic influence is best illustrated by demonstrating the effect of beta-antagonists on accommodative adaptation. Timolol induced a myopic shift in accommodative adaptation or "post-task tonic accommodation" by 0.33D to 0.44D relative to the control saline condition when assessed one minute following task completion (Gilmartin and Bullimore 1987, Rosenfield and Gilmartin 1987). The drug modified the regression pattern by prolonging the decay time to 50s, as compared with 20-30s for the control saline condition. This was especially evident for subjects exhibiting higher levels of pre-task tonic accommodation (Gilmartin and Bullimore 1987) (See Chapter 2). Moreover, in late-onset myopes, following a 45s near task, subjects exhibited a negative aftereffect or counter-adaptation of 0.50D which was significantly attenuated by application of a beta-antagonist (Rosenfield and Gilmartin 1989) (See Chapter 2). This suggested that the negative shift was related to the output of the adrenergic innervation. Since its regression was biased in a positive direction without any change in overall profile, this further suggested that the adrenergic component only influenced the magnitude of accommodative adaptation without modifying its time course. The inhibitory action of the sympathetic innervation on accommodative adaptation as evidenced by the preceding example lends credence to the speculation by

Gilmartin and Hogan (1985a) that the function of the inhibitory sympathetic component may be to counteract any accommodative adaptation or "hysteresis" that may be responsible for inducing nearwork-related myopia. From this, one can further speculate that a deficit in the sympathetic output may be a predisposing factor in generating abnormally greater amounts of nearpoint-induced transient myopia having a protracted time course, with this perhaps being exhibited in a more exaggerated form in certain population subgroups, such as symptomatic individuals who complain of transient blurred vision at distance following brief periods of nearwork (Ciuffreda and Ordoñez 1995). Also see Chapters 2 and 4.

SUMMARY

The sensory, motor, perceptual, anatomical, and pharmacological aspects of human accommodation are reviewed with emphasis on basic mechanisms. This information is critical to understand the more clinical aspects of accommodation with regard to myopigenesis.

REFERENCES

Alpern M. Accommodation. In: Davson H, (ed.), The eye, Vol. 3, New York: Academic Press; 1969; 217-54.

Biggs RD, Alpern M, Bennett DR. The effect of sympathomimetic drugs upon the amplitude of accommodation. Am J Ophthalmol. 1959; 48:169-72.

Bullimore M, Gilmartin B. Tonic accommodation, cognitive demand, and ciliary muscle innervation. Am J Optom Physiol Opt. 1987; 64:45-50.

Campbell FW. The minimum quantity of light required to elicit the accommodation reflex in man. J Physiol (Lond). 1954; 123:357-66.

Campbell FW. Correlation of accommodation between the two eyes. J Opt Soc Am. 1960; 50:738.

Campbell FW, Westheimer G. Dynamics of accommodation responses of the human eye. J Physiol. 1960; 151:285-95.

Campbell FW, Robson JG, Westheimer G. Fluctuations of accommodation under steady viewing conditions. J Physiol. 1959; 145:579-94.

Charman WN, Heron G. Fluctuations in accommodation: a review. Ophthal Physiol Opt. 1988; 8:1533-64.

Ciuffreda KJ. Accommodation and its anomalies. In: Charman WN, (ed.), Vision and visual dysfunction: visual optics and instrumentation, Vol. 1, London: MacMillan; 1991; 231-79.

Ciuffreda KJ. Accommodation, the pupil, and presbyopia. In: Benjamin J, Borish I (eds.), Clinical refraction: principles and practice: Philadelphia: Saunders, in press.

Ciuffreda KJ. Components of clinical near vergence testing. J Behav Optom. 1992; 3: 3-13.

Ciuffreda KJ, Kenyon RV. Accommodative vergence and accommodation in normals, amblyopes, and strabismics. In: Schor CM, Ciuffreda KJ (eds.), Vergence eye movements: basic and clinical aspects. Boston: Butterworths; 1983; 101-73.

Ciuffreda KJ, Kruger PK. Dynamics of human voluntary accommodation. Am J Optom Physiol Opt. 1988; 65:365-70.

Ciuffreda KJ, Ordoñez X. Abnormal transient myopia in symptomatic individuals after sustained nearwork. Optom Vis Sci. 1995; 72:506-10.

Ciuffreda KJ, Hokoda SC, Hung GK, Semmlow JL. Accommodative stimulus/response function in human amblyopia. Doc Ophthalmol. 1984; 56:303-26.

Cogan DG. Accommodation and the autonomic nervous system. Arch Ophthalmol. 1937; 18:739-66.

Dean AF. The relationship between response amplitude and contrast for cat striate cortical neurones. J Physiol. 1981; 318:413-227.

Fincham EF. The mechanism of accommodation. Br J Ophthalmol (Suppl). 1937; 8:5-80.

Fincham EF. The reflex reaction of accommodation. Trans Internat Opt Cong. 1951; 105-114.

Fisher SK, Ciuffreda KJ, Hammer S. Interocular equality of tonic accommodation and consensuality of accommodative hysteresis. Ophthal Physiol Opt. 1987; 7:17-20.

Fleming DG, Hall JL. Autonomic innervation of the ciliary body: a modified theory of accommodation. Am J Ophthalmol. 1959; 48:287-93.

Garner LF, Brown B, Baker R, Colgan M. The effect of phenylephrine hydrochloride on the resting point of accommodation. Invest Ophthalmol Vis Sci. 1983; 24:393-95.

Gilmartin B. A review of the role of sympathetic innervation of the ciliary muscle in ocular accommodation. Ophthal Physiol Opt. 1986; 6:23-37.

Gilmartin B, Bullimore MA. Sustained near-vision augments inhibitory sympathetic innervation of the ciliary muscle. Clin Vis Sci. 1987; 1:197-208.

Gilmartin B, Bullimore MA, Rosenfield M, Winn B, Owens H. Pharmacological effects on accommodative adaptation. Optom Vis Sci. 1992; 69:276-82.

Gilmartin B, Hogan RE.The relationship between tonic accommodation and ciliary muscle innervation. Invest Ophthalmol Vis Sci. 1985a; 26:1024-28.

Gilmartin B, Hogan RE. The role of the sympathetic nervous system in ocular accommodation and ametropia. Ophthal Physiol Opt. 1985b; 5:91-3.

Gilmartin B, Hogan RE, Thompson SM. The effect of timolol maleate on tonic accommodation, tonic vergence and pupil diameter. Invest Ophthal Vis Sci. 1984; 25:736-70.

Gullstrand A. Die optische abbildung in heterogenen medien die dioptrik der kristallinse des menschen. K Svenska Vetensk Akad Handl 1908; 43:1-58. Cited in Alpern M. Accommodation. In: Davson H, (ed.), The eye, Vol. 3, New York: Academic Press; 1969; 217-54.

Harrison RJ. Loss of fusional vergence with partial loss of accommodative convergence and accommodation following head injury. Bino Vis. 1987; 2:93-100.

Heath GG. Accommodative responses of totally color blind observers. Am J Optom Arch Am Acad Optom. 1956a; 33:457-65.

Heath GG. Components of accommodation. Am J Optom Arch Am Acad Optom. 1956b; 33:569-579.

Hung GK, Ciuffreda KJ. Dual-mode behavior in the human accommodation system. Ophthal Physiol Opt. 1988; 8:327-32.

Hung GK, Semmlow JL. Static behavior of accommodation and vergence: computer simulation of an interactive dual-feedback system. IEEE Trans Biomed Engn. 1980; BME-27:439-47.

Hurwitz BS, Davidowitz J, Chin NB, Breinin GB. The effects of the sympathetic nervous system on accommodation. I. Beta sympathetic nervous system. Arch Ophthalmol. 1972a; 87:668-74.

Hurwitz BS, Davidowitz J, Pachter BR, Breinin GB. The effects of the sympathetic nervous system on accommodation. II. Alpha sympathetic nervous system. Arch Ophthalmol. 1972b; 87:675-88.

Jaeger RJ, Benevento LA. A horseradish peroxidase study of the innervation of the internal structures of the eye. Invest Ophthalmol Vis Sci. 1980; 19:575-83.

Jampel RS. Representation of the near response on the cerebral cortex of the macaque. Am J Ophthalmol. 1959; 48:573-82.

Judge SJ, Cummings RG. Neurons in the monkey midbrain with activity related to vergence eye movement and accommodation. J Neurophysiol. 1986; 55:915-30.

Kaplan E, Shapley RM. X and Y cells in the lateral geniculate nucleus of macaque monkeys. J Physiol (Lond). 1982; 330:125-43.

Kotulak JC, Schor CM. A computational model of the error detector of human visual accommodation. Biol Cybern. 1986; 54:189-94.

Leibowitz HW, Owens DA. Night myopia and the intermediate dark focus of accommodation. J Opt Soc Am. 1975; 65:1121-28.

Leibowitz HW, Owens DA. New evidence for the intermediate position of relaxed accommodation. Doc Ophthalmol. 1978; 46:133-47.

Lograno MD, Reibaldi A. Receptor-responses in fresh human ciliary muscle. Br J Ophthalmol. 1986; 87:379-85.

Maddox EE. The clinical use of prisms. 2nd ed. Bristol: John Wright and Co.: 1893.

McCulloch C. The zonule of Zinn: its origin, course, and insertion, and its relation to neighboring strutures. Trans Am Ophthal Soc. 1954; 52:525-85.

Miege C, Denieul P. Mean response and oscillations of accommodation for various stimulus vergences in relation to accommodation feedback control. Ophthal Physiol Opt. 1988; 8:165-71.

Morgan MW. A new theory for the control of accommodation. Am J Optom Arch Am Acad Optom. 1946; 23:99-110.

Moses RA. Accommodation. In Moses RA, Hart WM, Jr., (eds.), Adler's physiology of the eye: clinical applications. St. Louis: The C.V. Mosby Co; 1987; 291-310.

Netter FH. Nervous system. In: The CIBA Collection of Medical Illustrations. vol. 1. New Jersey: CIBA. 1962; 92.

Ohtsuka K, Maekawa H, Takeda M, Uede N, Chiba S. Accommodation and convergence insufficiency with left middle cerebral artery occlusion. Am J Ophthalmol. 1988; 105:60-4.

Ong E, Ciuffreda KJ, Tannen B. Static accommodation in congenital nystagmus. Invest Ophthalmol Vis Sci. 1993; 34:194-204.

Phillips S, Shirachi D, Stark L. Analysis of accommodative response times using histogram information. Am J Optom Arch Am Acad Optom. 1972; 49:389-401.

Randle RJ, Murphy MR. The dynamic response of visual accommodation over a seven-day period. Am J Optom Physiol Opt. 1974; 51:530-44.

Rohen JW. Scanning electron microscopic studies of the zonular apparatus in human and monkey eyes. Invest Ophthalmol Vis Sci. 1979; 18:133-44.

Rosenfield M, Ciuffreda KJ, Hung GK, Gilmartin B. Tonic accommodation: a review. I. Basic aspects. Ophthal Physiol Opt. 1993; 13:266-84.

Rosenfield M, Gilmartin B. Oculomotor consequences of beta-adrenoceptor antagonism during sustained near vision. Ophthal Physiol Opt. 1987; 7:127-30.

Rosenfield M, Gilmartin B. Temporal aspects of accommodative adaptation. Optom Vis Sci. 1989; 66:229-34.

Rosenfield M, Gilmartin B, Cunningham E, Dattani N. The influence of alpha-adrenergic agents on tonic accommodation. Curr Eye Res. 1990; 9:267-72.

Salzmann M. The anatomy and histology of the human eyeball in the normal state: its development and senescence. trans. Brown EVL. Chicago: The University of Chicago Press. 1912; 111-5.

Schnider CM, Ciuffreda KJ, Cooper J, Kruger PB. Accommodation dynamics in divergence excess exotropia. Invest Ophthalmol Vis Sci. 1984; 25:414-8.

Shirachi D, Liu J, Lee M, Jang J, Wang J, Stark L. Accommodation dynamics. I. Range nonlinearity. Am J Optom Physiol Opt. 1978; 55:631-41.

Stark L. Presbyopia in light of accommodation. Am J Optom Physiol Opt. 1988; 65: 407-16.

Stephens KG. Effect of the sympathetic nervous system on accommodation. Am J Optom Physiol Opt. 1985; 62:402-6.

Toates FM. Accommodation function of the human eye. Physiol Rev. 1972; 52:828-63.

Tornqvist G. The relative importance of the parasympathetic and sympathetic nervous systems for accommodation in monkeys. Invest Ophthalmol Vis Sci. 1967; 6:612-7.

Van Alphen GWHM. The adrenergic receptors of the intraocular muscles of the human eye. Invest Ophthalmol. 1976; 15:502-5.

Wax MB, Molinoff PB. Distribution and properties of beta-adrenergic receptors in humans iris-ciliary body. Invest Ophthalmol Vis Sci. 1987; 28:420-30.

Weale RA. A biography of the eye. London: HK Lewis Ltd; 1982.

Winn B, Pugh JR, Gilmartin B, Owens H. Arterial pulse modulates steady-state ocular accommodation. Curr Eye Res. 1990; 9:971-5.

Wyatt HJ. Some aspects of the mechanics of accommodation. Vis Res. 1988; 28:75-86.

Young T. On the mechanism of the eye. Phil Trans. 1801; 91:23-88.

Zetterstrom C. The effect of phenylephrine on the accommodative process in man. Acta Ophthalmol. 1984; 62:872-8.

Zetterstrom C. The effects of thymoxamine, phenylephrine and cyclopentolate on the accommodative process in man. Acta Ophthalmol. 1987; 65:699-704.

Zetterstrom C. Effects of adrenergic drugs on accommodation and distant refraction in daylight and darkness: a laseroptometric study. Acta Ophthalmol. 1988; 66:58-64.

Zetterstrom C, Hahnenberger R. Pharmacological characterization of human ciliary muscle adrenoceptors in vitro. Exp Eye Res. 1988; 46:421-30.

CHAPTER 2 ACCOMMODATION AND REFRACTIVE GROUP

Over the years, accommodation has been implicated in the development and progression of myopia. This has involved anatomical, physiological, sensory, motor, perceptual, and biomechanical aspects. In addition, some have suggested that accommodation per se is abnormal in myopes, with this also contributing to their myopia. Thus, the intent of this chapter is to provide a critical and detailed review regarding the various components of accommodation as a function of refractive group to serve as a basis for subsequent related discussions in the book.

STATIC ACCOMMODATION

Steady-State Accommodative Response

Studies investigating accommodation as a function of refractive state predominantly used binocular near tasks, so that blur and disparity-induced accommodation both contributed to the aggregate response (along with proximal and tonic accommodation to a small extent). Accommodation was assessed using either an infrared or a laser optometer. The results from the majority of studies suggested that the accommodative stimulus/response function or profile varied slightly with refractive state, with the most common trend being hyperopes, followed by emmetropes and myopes, having progressively decreasing slope values (Table 2-1) (Ramsdale 1979, McBrien and Millodot 1986b, Rosenfield and Gilmartin 1987c, Rosenfield and Gilmartin 1988c, Jones 1990, Bullimore et al. 1992, Gwiazda et al. 1993, 1995a). In contrast, other studies found no significant accommodative difference under certain conditions between refractive groups (Table 2-1) (Ramsdale 1985, Rosenfield and Gilmartin 1987a, Tokoro 1988, Bullimore et al. 1992, Gwiazda et al. 1993). This can be gleaned from a composite graph of the available static and dynamic results in the literature on accommodation for the different refractive groups (Figure 2-1).

One of the most cited studies that demonstrated a refraction-dependent accommodative profile was by McBrien and Millodot (1986b). The study showed that hyperopes exhibited the highest slopes (0.97), followed by emmetropes (0.92), early-onset myopes (0.88), and late-onset myopes (0.87). However, no statistical analysis was performed to demonstrate that

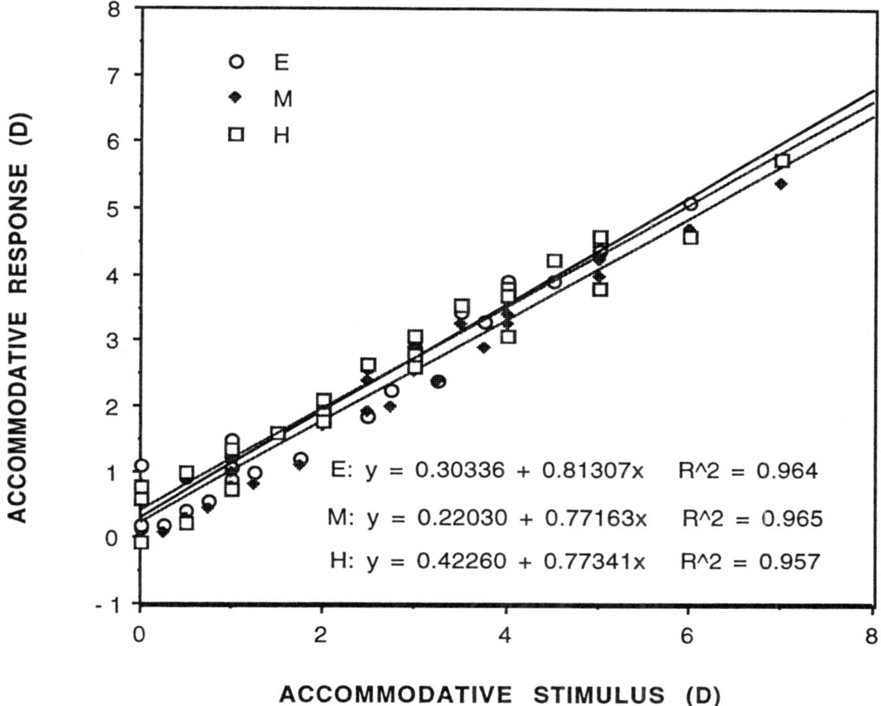

Figure 2-1: Summary graph of accommodation as a function of refractive group from the literature, where E= emmetropes, M= myopes, and H= hyperopes.

these slope differences were significant, and thus this still remains an open question. The presumed slope difference among the refractive groups was mainly due to differences in accommodative lags, particularly at the higher stimulus levels. Statistically significant differences between most refractive groups were found only at stimulus levels of 4 and 5D. Late-onset myopes exhibited the greatest lag (0.64 to 0.83D), followed by early-onset myopes (0.56 to 0.69D), emmetropes (0.35 to 0.54D) and hyperopes (0.30 to 0.38D) in decreasing order with the maximum average lag difference between groups being 0.45D. A significant correlation of 0.5 was found between refractive status and the accommodative response gradient, although the r^2 value (0.25) was quite low. Overall, the study demonstrated that the response functions of the different refractive groups followed more or less the typical shape of the accommodative stimulus/response function, although the expected "lead of accommodation" characterizing responses for lower stimulus levels was either absent or very small. This was addressed by the authors as being the consequence of the calibration of the autorefractor. It

TABLE 2-1:
SUMMARY RESULTS OF STEADY-STATE ACCOMMODATION AS A FUNCTION OF REFRACTIVE GROUP

INVESTIGATOR (YEAR)	DIAGNOSTIC CATEGORIES	N	AGES (yrs)	APPARATUS/ VIEWING CONDITION	TARGET/ DISTANCE	RESULTS
Ramsdale (1979)	E (±0.50 sph) H M	>10	18-31	laser optometer/monocular	Snellen 6/6 @+2 to-7 in 1D steps	E>M,H
Ramsdale (1985)	E (±0.50 sph & <1 cyl) H (+0.50 to +5.50 sph & <1 cyl) M (-0.50 sph to -7.75 & <1 cyl)	40	18-34	laser optometer/binocular	Snellen E 6/3-6/9 @ 0-5 D sph (in 0.50 steps)	E=H= M
McBrien & Millodot (1986b)	E (-0.25 to +0.74 sph & ≤1 cyl) H (+0.74 sph & ≤1 cyl) EOM (>-0.25 sph, ≤1cyl & ≤13y onset) LOM (>-0.25 sph, ≤1cyl & ≥15y onset)	40	18-23	infrared optometer/binocular	1.5' @ 20, 25, 33, 50, 100, 200 & 600 cm	H>E>EOM>LOM
Rosenfield & Gilmartin (1987a)	E (± 0.50 sph & ≤ 0.50cyl) EOM (>-0.50sph & <15y onset) LOM (>-0.50 sph & ≥15y onset)	51	~21	infrared optometer/binocular	N6 @ 33cm, 3.9 & 4.6D	EOM=LOM
Rosenfield & Gilmartin (1987c)	E ($\bar{x}$ = ±0.10 sph) EOM ($\bar{x}$= -3.92sph & <15y onset) LOM ($\bar{x}$= -1.71sph & >15y onset)	45	~22	infrared optometer/binocular	letters in Badal system @ 2.50 & 3.25D	LOM>E>EOM
Rosenfield & Gilmartin (1988c)	E (± 0.50 sph & ≤0.50 cyl) LOM (-0.75 to -4 sph & ≥15y onset)	20	~21	infrared optometer/binocular	N6 numbers @ 33 cm	E>LOM
Tokoro (1988)	E M (<-3.50 sph & <1cyl)	16	20-35	infrared optometer/monocular	cross target @ 20cm to 2m	accommodative lag @ 5D: E=M

Jones (1990)	E (-0.25 to +0.75 sph) M (-1.25 to -3.50 sph)	48	N.A.	objective infrared device	0 to 3D	slope:E>M
Bullimore, Gilmartin & Royston (1992)	E (plano to ±0.50 sph & ≤0.25 cyl) LOM (-0.50 & -3.50 sph & >15y onset)	28	19-23	infrared optometer/binocular	numbers (24') @ 100, 33 & 20 cm	Passive: E>LOM Active: E=LOM
Gwiazda, Thorn, Bauer & Held (1993)	E (-0.25 to +0.50 sph eq. & ≤1 cyl) new M (-0.50 to -6.25 sph eq. & ≤1 cyl)	64	5-17	infrared optometer/monocular	20/30 &20/100 letters @ 0.25 to 4m in 7 steps or lenses (0 to ± 4 sph in 0.50D steps)	real space:E>M w/minus lens:E>>M w/plus lens:E=M
Gwiazda, Bauer, Thorn & Held (1995a)	E (+0.75 to -0.25sph & ≤1 cyl) M (-0.38 to -5.25 sph & ≤1 cyl)	63	6-18	infrared optometer/monocular	20/100 letters @ 4 m with plano to -10D sph (in 0.5 or 1D steps)	slope: E>M

Key: Symbols for this and all other similar tables are:

M= myopes
E= emmetropes
H= hyperopes
LOM= late-onset myopes
EOM= early-onset myopes
sph= sphere
cyl= cylinder
sph eq= spherical equivalent

D= diopter; unit for refractive diagnostic conditions
BO= base-out prisms
pl= plano
TA= tonic accommodation
N.A.= not available

might also be due to the open-field nature of the optometer used, thus minimizing the effects of proximal accommodation (Rosenfield et al. 1993). In addition, even though the accommodative response gradients encompassed a range well within normal limits, nonetheless, the overall accommodative gains were somewhat higher in comparison to those found by other investigators (Mordi 1991, Ong et al. 1991). This can probably be attributed to the binocular paradigm used in their study which invoked the addition of convergence accommodation.

McBrien and Millodot (1986b) explained the difference in accommodative response between refractive groups based on Charman's idea (1982), which implicated tonic accommodation as the "point of equilibrium" between parasympathetic and sympathetic innervation; the former was believed responsible for "positive" or increased accommodation, and the latter was believed responsible for "negative" or decreased accommodation, relative to this "equilibrium" position. Myopia was suggested to be due to a weak sympathetic/strong parasympathetic innervation. This would lead to a reduced accommodative range, particularly over the sympathetic region, which would adversely affect distant vision and thereby render the subject myopic.

However, the above ideas are not in agreement with other studies. Firstly, negative accommodation is not solely sympathetically-mediated; hence, a reduced sympathetic range is not equivalent to myopia. Secondly, the sympathetic system is too slow to drive the standard far-to-near and near-to-far accommodative dynamics. Finally, a weak sympathetic/strong parasympathetic innervation is not supported by Tornqvist's pharmacological evidence (1967). According to his findings, the degree of sympathetic innervation was related with the concurrent parasympathetic background activity.

A study by Rosenfield and Gilmartin (1988c) presented results that appeared to be consistent with the above findings. When late-onset myopes were presented with a 3D target, they exhibited a small but significantly lower accommodative response as compared with emmetropes. Mean differences of approximately 0.10 to 0.55D were observed.

Similarly, Bullimore et al. (1992) found refractive group differences in within-task accommodative response as a function of the accommodative task. A Canon Autoref R-1 infrared optometer was used to assess the accommodative response of emmetropes and late-onset myopes at 3 dioptric stimulus levels (1, 3 and 5D). The experimental paradigm consisted of two binocular viewing conditions differentiated by the requisite level of mental effort or cognitive load: (1) a passive condition, wherein the subject was simply instructed to read a matrix of numbers to himself, and (2) an active condition, wherein the subject was asked to add up each set of numbers. The difference in accommodative response between the two conditions varied with refractive group as well as accommodative demand. In emmetropes, the cognitively-induced change in accommodation was stimulus-dependent. A significant increase in accommodative response was found only for the 1D stimulus level, while a slight reduction in response was reported for the 5D stimulus level. In contrast, the imposition of a higher cognitive demand consistently induced increased accommodation for late-onset myopes at all stimulus levels. According to the authors, this response profile was comparable to those obtained on emmetropes for high stimulus levels when sympatholytic agents were administered (Bullimore and Gilmartin 1988). Further data analyses whereby the accommodative responses between the two refractive groups were compared indicated that under the active condition, accommodation between the two refractive groups was equivalent. On the other hand, under the passive condition, emmetropes accommodated significantly greater than late-onset myopes, although the mean difference amounted to only 0.13D and was only observed for the 5D stimulus level. The authors suggested that the reduced accommodation characterizing late-onset myopes may reflect their increased tolerance to blur due to their habitually poor distant vision in the early years when they were uncorrected. They also suggested that it might be an indication of a difference in the accommodation and vergence relationship.

The aforementioned studies primarily used a binocular paradigm. Hence, the measured accommodative response included input from vergence accommodation. Unfortunately, this confounds comparison with monocular blur-driven studies as well as complicates the interpretation of results, since the drive from vergence accommodation as well as its interactions with blur-driven accommodation must now be considered. In light of this, it is desirable to investigate the monocular accommodative response to delineate the contribution of blur alone for the different refractive groups. Recently, Gwiazda et al. (1993) investigated the monocular accommodative responses in emmetropic and newly myopic children (Figure 2-2). The accommodative stimulus was altered using either a moveable target in free space or with plus or minus lenses and a fixed target at near in free space. The use of spherical lenses produced reduced slopes, with the effect being more pronounced with negative lenses. Emmetropes consistently showed a significantly higher slope relative to the early-onset myopes under both the moveable target conditions (0.88 versus 0.78) and negative lens conditions (0.61 versus 0.20). However, positive lenses revealed no difference in slopes between the emmetropes (0.69) and the myopes (0.64). The authors suggested that their findings reflected the reduced blur appreciation in early-onset myopes, with the qualification that it was directionally-sensitive. However, there are some methodological concerns. First, accommodation

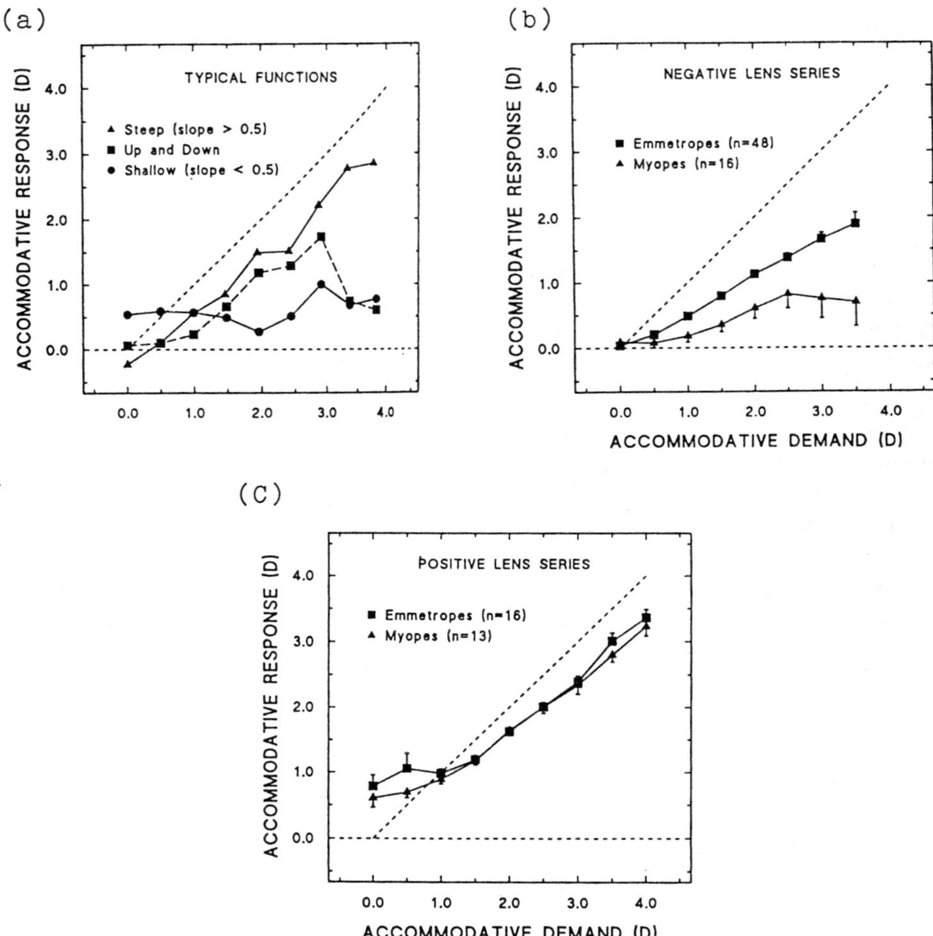

Figure 2-2 : (a) Typical accommodative response functions. The steep slope is characteristic of emmetropic eyes; the shallow and the up and down are characteristic of myopic eyes. (b) Accommodative responses shown by myopic (▲) and emmetropic (■) eyes to a 4.0-m target (a 3 x 3 array of 20/100 letters) viewed through a series of negative lenses. Error bars represent the standard error of the mean for each data point. (c) Accommodative responses shown by myopic (▲) and emmetropic (■) eyes to a 0.25-m target (a 3 x 3 array of 20/100 letters) viewed through a series of positive lenses. Error bars represent the standard error of the mean for each data point (Reprinted with permission, Gwiazda et al. 1993).

as measured with the autorefractor was taken with corrective spectacle lenses in front of the subject's eye. The lenses were positioned with a pantoscopic tilt of 15 deg. As a result, the spherical power was altered, and some astigmatism was induced. In fact, the authors acknowledged the existence of this problem, and reported that tilting of the lenses resulted in a 6% average reduction of accommodative demand. However, no compensation for the induced error was incorporated into the final results. It appears, at least under the moveable target condition, that this artificially induced dioptric error could explain in part the reduced responsivity in early-onset myopes. Secondly, since the subject population consisted of children who did not have a cycloplegic refraction performed, it is possible that a miscategorization in refractive status occurred, especially with respect to hyperopes versus emmetropes.

Overall, the majority of studies suggests that steady-state accommodative responsivity at both far and intermediate near distances is related to refractive status. Myopes appear to exhibit reduced accommodation, with these changes occurring more or less concurrent with the development of myopia (Gwiazda et al. 1995a). See Chapter 7. Possible explanations that have been proposed regarding the reduced accommodative responsivity in myopes have included the following:

(1) Myopes have reduced blur appreciation or increased blur tolerance as suggested in the data presented by both Bullimore et al. (1992) and Gwiazda et al. (1993). In other words, this translates into an effectively increased depth-of-focus. The increased threshold for blur detection appears to be exaggerated in cases of negative lens-induced blur (Gwiazda et al. 1993). This characteristic suggests that myopes may be unable to use pure blur cues effectively, and hence, may have to make use of other cues such as disparity or proximity for reinforcement. However, open-loop proximally-induced accommodation in late-onset myopes was found to be, on the contrary, less than that found in emmetropes (Rosenfield and Gilmartin 1990), and thus this would be of minimal assistance. (See section on proximal accommodation.) And, while open-loop convergent accommodation was similar across refractive groups (Rosenfield and Gilmartin 1988b, Jones 1990), closed-loop disparity-induced accommodation was greater for myopes versus emmetropes (Rosenfield and Gilmartin 1987c, Rosenfield and Gilmartin 1988c), and thus could be of value. However, the contribution from disparity-induced accommodation is apparently not sufficient, since accommodative responses for myopes are still reduced. However, while increased blur tolerance is a plausible mechanism to explain the reduced accommodation, it is unclear why the subjective response to positive and negative lens-induced defocus should differ. Further work in this area is clearly needed. For example, the subjective depth-of-focus as a function of refractive group should be assessed carefully to determine directly if blur sensitivity is reduced in myopes in particular.

(2) Myopes may possess deficient accommodative gain (Jones 1990). Taking it one step further, one could speculate that the reduced gain may be either neural or biomechanical in nature. A neurally-based decrease would

suggest reduced innervation, while a biomechanically-based decrease would suggest involvement of the peripheral apparatus including the crystalline lens, ciliary muscle, and zonules. In fact, biometric investigations have revealed flatter and lower powered crystalline lenses in myopes (Stenstrom 1948, Francois and Goes 1969, Garner et al. 1992). Storey and Rabie (1983) further suggested that myopes accommodated “less efficiently” due to the greater crystalline lens change induced in myopes per diopter of change in accommodative stimulus. On the other hand, Sato (1957) suggested hypertrophy of the ciliary muscle as a consequence of overexertion from increased near work demand, and this would be counter to the notion of reduced gain. If anything, under this scenario the gain might be expected to fall on the high normal side. Such a hypothesis clearly needs to be tested.

(3) A difference in the accommodative-vergence relationship between refractive groups might exist (Bullimore et al. 1992). Previous data on accommodative vergence showed that myopes possessed higher AC/A ratios than emmetropes (Manas 1955, Flom and Takahashi 1962), and early-onset myopes had greater AC/A ratios than late-onset myopes and emmetropes (Rosenfield and Gilmartin 1987a). Data regarding convergent accommodation and disparity-induced accommodation have been discussed earlier, and this will be considered later in this chapter with respect to refractive groups. Further elucidation in this area may be obtained by separately investigating each of the accommodative components.

Amplitude of Accommodation

The accommodative amplitude represents the maximum accommodative response capable of being elicited by the system. It is taken as the reciprocal of the closest distance from the subject’s ocular plane of refraction (calculated from the eye’s principal planes, or more practically, from the corneal apex) at which an object can still be seen clearly (discounting the depth-of-focus) (Ciuffreda, in press). Clinically, it is usually assessed monocularly and binocularly by the push-up technique (Borish 1970). Mean clinical values obtained from the normal population are age-dependent (Duane 1912), with the amplitude decreasing from a maximum at age 5 years or so (Ciuffreda, in press) to a minimum of zero at age 52 years or so (Hamasaki et al. 1956) at a rate of approximately 0.3D/year (Hoffstetter 1944).

The results, as well as the more important details of various investigations that measured amplitude of accommodation as a function of refractive state, are tabulated in Table 2-2. The most common method of amplitude measurement was the monocular push-up technique using a near point rule. The mean amplitudes reported for the different studies were generally consistent with the accepted norms for the specific age ranges of the subjects (Duane 1912). The only exception was the study by Fisher et al. (1987),

TABLE 2-2:SUMMARY RESULTS OF ACCOMMODATIVE AMPLITUDE AS A FUNCTION OF REFRACTIVE GROUP

INVESTIGATOR (YEAR)	DIAGNOSTIC CATEGORIES	N	AGES (yrs.)	TECHNIQUE	RESULTS
Turner (1958)	E (± 0.75 sph); H (> +0.75 sph); M (> -0.75 sph)	~1000 eyes	<13 to >67 inclusive	monocular push-up	<30y:inconclusive >35y: M=E=H
Baldwin (1965)	EOM ($\bar{x}$= 2.97 sph eq)	80	$\bar{x}$= 27	N.A.	EOM= general population
Fledelius (1981)	E (plano to - 0.90 sph); H (≥ +1 sph); juvenile M (>-0.90sph w/mean onset @11.5y)	137	18	monocular push-up	M>E>H
Maddock, Millodot, Leat & Johnson (Davis) (1981)	E (plano); low M (<-3 sph); high M(>-3 sph)	40	-25	measured with laser optometer	low M>E; high M=low M; high M=E
Gawron (1981)	E (plano to -1 sph); M (>-1 sph); H (≤+0.25 sph)	152	17-28	push-up	M=E=H
McBrien & Millodot (1986a)	E; H; EOM (≤13 y); LOM (≥15 y)	80	18-22	monocular push-up	LOM>EOM>E>H>
Fisher, Ciuffreda & Levine (1987)	E (± 0.75 sph); H (+0.75 sph); low M (>-0.75 but ≤ -4 sph); high M (>-4sph)	48	21-35	monocular push-up with reduced Snellen in Badal system using Hartinger optometer	E=H=lowM=highM
Zhai & Guan (1988)	E (-0.25 to +0.50 sph) M (-1 to -3 sph & ≤0.5cyl)	128	10-19	dynamic accommodo-polyrecorder	E>M
Gwiazda, Bauer, Thorn & Held (1995a)	E (+0.75 to -0.25 sph & ≤ 1cyl) M (-0.38 to -5.25 sph & ≤ 1cyl)	63	6-18	monocular with minus lens (0 to 10D) & array of letters at 4m using infrared optometer	E>M

which reported a somewhat depressed overall amplitude of approximately 6D. Equally reduced amplitudes were also evident for the individual refractive groups. The subject population comprised an age range from 21-35 years. It appears that their broad and unequal subject age distribution might have resulted in the overall decreased amplitude; this might have also contributed to the reduced likelihood of detecting any differences between refractive groups.

Despite the fact that the mean amplitudes reported by most other studies were comparable to that of Duane (1912), a few demonstrated an extremely wide range of values. These studies exhibited increased variability in the order of ±2-4D (1 standard deviation), thereby rendering values which exceeded both the higher and lower limits of Duane's curve (Fledelius 1981, Maddock et al. 1981, Gawron 1981). For example, Fledelius (1981) reported an age-appropriate mean accommodative amplitude (10.7-13.8D) within the limits set by Duane (10.1D-14.4D). However, the range of amplitudes was considerably larger. These were: 6.3-16.7D, 6.6-14.8D and 8.3-22.2D for emmetropes, hyperopes and juvenile myopes, respectively. To compound the problem, it appears that the data reported by Fledelius referred to ocular accommodation, whereas Duane reported spectacle accommodation. Thus, the latter data would be artificially inflated with respect to the former. This would further exaggerate any discrepancies between the studies.

The results of the studies on accommodative amplitude as a function of refractive state are equivocal (Table 2-2). Approximately one-half found no significant difference between refractive groups (Turner 1958, Baldwin 1965, Gawron 1981, Maddock et al. 1981, Fisher et al. 1987). The other half reported either a significantly increased amplitude in myopes followed by emmetropes and then hyperopes, in decreasing order (Fledelius 1981, Maddock et al. 1981, McBrien and Millodot 1986a) (Figure 2-3), or the reverse trend (Zhai and Guan 1988, Gwiazda et al. 1995a). The differences between these studies may be attributed to several factors, one of which may be the characteristics of the comparison group. For example, Baldwin (1965) compared the accommodative amplitude of his myopic subjects to those reported for the general population. The latter consists of ametropes, including myopes, which would bias the accommodative amplitude values and therefore might not represent a valid population for comparative purposes. Another factor as indicated earlier is the age distribution. It is interesting to note that in those studies in which no amplitude difference was demonstrated, the ages of the subject population encompassed at least an entire decade. Since the accommodative amplitude is age-dependent, and the maximum differential amplitude between refractive groups appears to be relatively small and inconsistent, if at all present, with a difference in

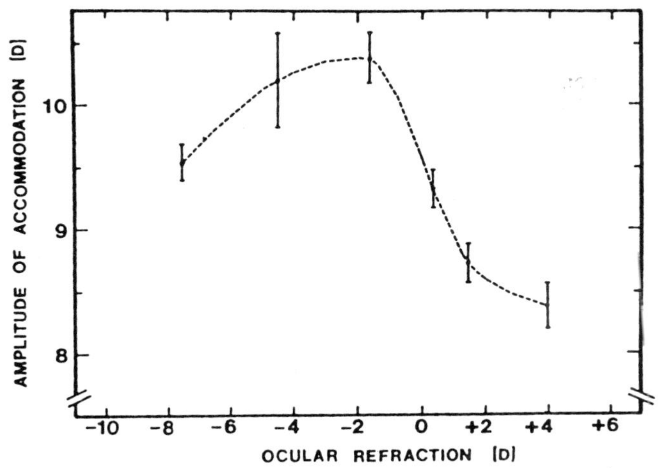

Figure 2-3 : The relationship between amplitude of accommodation and ocular refraction for 80 subjects. Each point represents the mean amplitude of accommodation for subjects falling within the following ranges of refraction: -9.00D to -6.00D; -5.99D to -3.00D; -2.99D to -0.26D; -0.25D to +0.75D; +0.76D to +3.00D; and +3.01D to +6.00D. The error bars represent ± 1 SEM (Reprinted with permission, McBrien and Millodot 1986a).

mean amplitude ranging from only 1-3 diopters, the findings of some may be contaminated by the use of such a wide age distribution across refractive group. Moreover, age distribution may have also played a role in the other two studies which demonstrated a greater accommodative amplitude for emmetropes. In these aforementioned studies, the subjects used were somewhat younger in age.

In addition, discrepancies between the various studies may also be explained by methodological differences. Some assessed monocular accommodative amplitude by moving the target along the median line. McBrien and Millodot (1986a) addressed this issue and have thus taken the angular distance from the visual axis into account when computing the true target-to-eye distance for the final accommodative amplitude, while Turner (1958) indicated that compensated differences for data falling below 8D can safely be ignored since it amounted to only 0.25D. Hence, no correction factor was applied to his set of data. Aside from the above, it is not clear whether two other studies (Fledelius 1981, Gawron 1981) moved the target along the line-of-sight or the median line. The procedure of moving the target along the median plane may pose other problems. It will introduce versional eye movements. Extreme lateral gaze has been shown to affect the amplitude of accommodation. For example, adduction by as much as 40 degrees increased the accommodative amplitude by approximately 1D (Ripple 1952). It is not known, however, if this effect varies uniformly across refractive groups. Furthermore, the type of target used for the assessment of amplitude may also pose a problem. Most studies used real targets that were moved in physical space. However, the target used by Fisher et al. (1987) consisted of a reduced Snellen chart incorporated into a Badal system. The absence of proximal cues might explain, in part, their findings of lowered overall amplitudes. In fact, the study by Gwiazda et al. (1995a) used a fixed target, while the accommodative stimulus change was introduced through the use of spherical lenses. This technique similarly yielded reduced accommodative amplitude values. In addition to the problems stated above, it is not clear from some of the studies using hyperopes whether or not a cycloplegic refraction had been performed. If not, any uncorrected or latent hyperopia would mask itself as an apparent decrease in the measured amplitude. Following along the same lines, it is important to reiterate that comparison between the different studies is hindered by the fact that some studies reported ocular accommodation, others spectacle accommodation, while the rest failed to specify this important reference point.

Lastly, it should be mentioned that the near point values reported by Gawron (1981) do not accurately represent accommodative amplitude. Since corrective lenses were not worn during any of the measurements, the reported near points appeared to have included the uncorrected ametropic value as well. Hence, the measured amplitude for the myopes would be artificially inflated and vice versa for the hyperopes. We have therefore taken the accommodative range, which the author defined as the difference between the far point and near point, as the true amplitude. However, a problem may still arise in cases of uncorrected astigmatism in young subjects with full accommodative ability.

The exact mechanism underlying the finding of differences in accommodative amplitude between refractive groups remains unknown. In an attempt to explain their result of higher accommodative amplitudes in myopes, McBrien and Millodot (1986a) put forth two possible explanations:

1) They attributed it to the weak sympathetic/strong parasympathetic facility associated with myopia as postulated by Charman (1982). They claimed that the strong parasympathetic innervation would lead to a higher accommodative amplitude. However, this runs contrary to their other study on accommodative stimulus/ response function as discussed earlier (McBrien and Millodot 1986b).
2) In direct contrast to the above but in line with Tornqvist's pharmacological evidence (1967), McBrien and Millodot (1986a) suggested that myopes may have reduced autonomic innervation. According to Tornqvist, the magnitude of the sympathetic inhibitory effect is dependent upon the underlying parasympathetic level. Therefore, based on this, myopes have weak parasympathetic as well as weak sympathetic facilities (McBrien and Millodot 1986a). Accordingly, a reduced sympathetically-mediated inhibition would be in effect. As a consequence, the parasympathetic facility would be left uninhibited. This might then explain the higher accommodative amplitude observed in myopes. How-

ever, this too is contrary to their ideas as discussed earlier for the accommodative stimulus/response function.

Convergent/Disparity-induced Accommodation

Convergent accommodation refers to that accommodation elicited by retinal disparity by way of the synkinetic link from disparity vergence to the accommodative system. It is assessed with blur-driven accommodation rendered open-loop, i.e.without visual feedback regarding blur of the retinal image. Convergent-accommodation may be differentiated from disparity-induced accommodation, the latter of which is measured under closed-loop conditions, i.e., with normal visual feedback regarding retinal blur, with accommodation now being driven primarily by both disparity and blur (Rosenfield and Gilmartin 1987c, Ciuffreda 1992, Hung et al. 1994).

Convergent Accommodation (Table 2-3)

Rosenfield and Gilmartin (1988b) assessed convergent accommodation in three age-matched refractive groups: emmetropes, early-onset myopes (onset ≥15 years of age) and late-onset myopes (onset <15 years of age). Target distances were 33 and 100 cm. Accommodation was measured objectively with a Canon R-1 infrared optometer. Small amounts of disparity were introduced using 3 and 6 prism diopters of base-out prisms (total) to provide slight to moderate non-congruent conditions (Footnote). The accommodative system was rendered open-loop with either 0.5 mm pinholes before the eyes or with a target consisting of a 0.1mm spot of light. There was no refractive group difference in convergent-accommodation for either the two target distances or the disparity stimuli. Mean CA/C ratio values for the three refractive groups ranged from 0.34 to 0.41D per meter angle, which were consistent with other studies (Hung and Semmlow 1980, Schor and Kotulak 1986, Tsuetaki and Schor 1987). And, no significant refractive group difference in the CA/C ratio was found. Likewise, using a similar range of vergence stimuli, Jones (1990) failed to elicit any significant difference in the CA/C ratio between emmetropes and myopes. However, the maximum prism used in both studies was only 6 prism diopters, equivalent to approximately 1 meter angle of additional disparity vergence stimulation, and thus only moderate target non-congruence was present. A larger range of prism values might have elicited a difference between groups, as well as provided a better estimate of the CA/C ratio, since one is essentially using linear regression to obtain this value.

This absence of a difference is supported in a more recent longitudinal study by Jiang (1995). In this study, the CA/C ratios of 44 young adult subjects were determined. This was performed at 6-month intervals over the course of two to three years. Accommodation was assessed objectively with a Canon R-1 infrared optometer, while subjects binocularly viewed a single pixel dimly displayed on a computer screen. The target was presented at three different distances: 2, 1 and 0.5m. Subjects were classified into four refractive groups. Subjects who exhibited a mean spherical equivalent refractive error in the range of +0.37 to -0.25D were classified as emmetropes, while those whose refractive error were at least -0.37D and characterized by a progressive nature were categorized as late-onset myopes. The "onset" group consisted of emmetropes who developed myopia exceeding -0.50D at the conclusion of the study. No significant differences in CA/C ratios were found between any of the refractive groups. From all of the above studies, there appears to be no refractive-error based difference in the CA/C ratio. However, a wider range of vergence stimulation would be highly desirable.

Disparity-induced Accommodation (Table 2-4)

In an investigation of disparity-induced accommodation as a function of refractive group, Rosenfield and Gilmartin (1987c) studied static accommodative and vergence interactions under closed-loop conditions in a population consisting of emmetropes, early-onset myopes (onset<15 years of age) and late-onset myopes (onset >15 years of age). A Canon R-1 infrared optometer was used to measure ocular accommodation objectively. Targets consisted of high-contrast letters. The disparity stimulus was introduced by the addition of a 4 prism diopter (p.d.) base-out prism, and the blur stimulus was introduced by varying target vergence within a Badal system to produce either 2.50 D or 3.25 D accommodative stimulus levels, thus yielding 4 non-congruent accommodation and vergence stimulus conditions: 2.50 D/ 0 p.d., 2.50 D/ 4 p.d., 3.25 D/ 0 p.d. and 3.25 D/ 4 p.d., which were varied in a pseudorandom manner. Disparity-induced accommodation was calculated as the difference in accommodation between the 0 and 4 p.d. condition for each accommodative stimulus level. Results showed that statistically higher disparity-induced accommodative values were found for late-onset myopes as compared to both the early-onset myopes and emmetropes (Figure 2-4). Initial disparity-induced accommodative values at the 2.50D level were 0.37D, 0.19D and 0.21D for late-onset myopes, early-onset myopes and emmetropes, respectively, and 0.26D, 0.27D and 0.11D at the 3.25D stimulus level for these same refractive groups. The generally small and relatively inconsistent differences found between refractive groups could probably be attributed to the use of non-congruent, non-naturalistic disparity and blur stimuli. Furthermore, such modest levels of non-congruence make expected differences small, perhaps leading to its lack of repeatability. The authors suggested that the general finding of higher disparity-induced accommodation in late-onset myopes could be attributed

TABLE 2-3:SUMMARY RESULTS OF CONVERGENT ACCOMMODATION AS A FUNCTION OF REFRACTIVE GROUP

INVESTIGATOR (YEAR)	DIAGNOSTIC CATEGORIES	N	AGES (yrs.)	APPARATUS	TARGET/DISTANCE	RESULTS
Rosenfield & Gilmartin (1988b)	E (± 0.50 sph & ≤0.50 cyl) EOM (>-0.50 sph & <15y onset) LOM (>-0.50 sph & ≥15y onset)	30	~23	infrared optometer	1) 0.1mm spot of light @ 33 cm & 100cm 2) N6 letters with 0.5mm pinhole @ 33 cm; both with 0, 3 & 6 BO prism	E=EOM=LOM
Jones (1990)	E (+0.75 to -0.25 sph) M (-1.25 to -3.50 sph)	48	N.A.	infrared optometer	4BI to 6BO prism diopters	E=M
Jiang (1995)	E (+0.37 to -0.25 sph eq) LOM (≤-0.37 sph eq) onset (E who developed myopia >–0.50sph eq)	44	18-27	infrared optometer	dim 0.5' pixel @ 2,1&0.5m	E= onset= LOM

TABLE 2-4: SUMMARY RESULTS OF DISPARITY-INDUCED ACCOMMODATION AS A FUNCTION OF REFRACTIVE GROUP

INVESTIGATOR (YEAR)	DIAGNOSTI C CATEGORIES	N	AGES (yrs.)	APPARATUS	TARGET/DISTANCE	RESULTS
Rosenfield & Gilmartin (1987c)	E ($\bar{x}$ = ± 0.10 sph) EOM ($\bar{x}$ = -3.92 sph & <15y onset) LOM ($\bar{x}$ = -1.71sph & >15y onset)	45	~22	infrared optometer	letters in a Badal system @ 2.50 & 3.25D sph with 0 & 4 BO prism	LOM>EOM,E
Rosenfield & Gilmartin (1988c)	E (± 0.50 sph & ≤0.50cyl) LOM (range -0.75 to -4 sph & ≥15y onset)	20	~21	infrared optometer	N6 numbers @ 33c m with 0, 3 & 6 BO prism	LOM>E

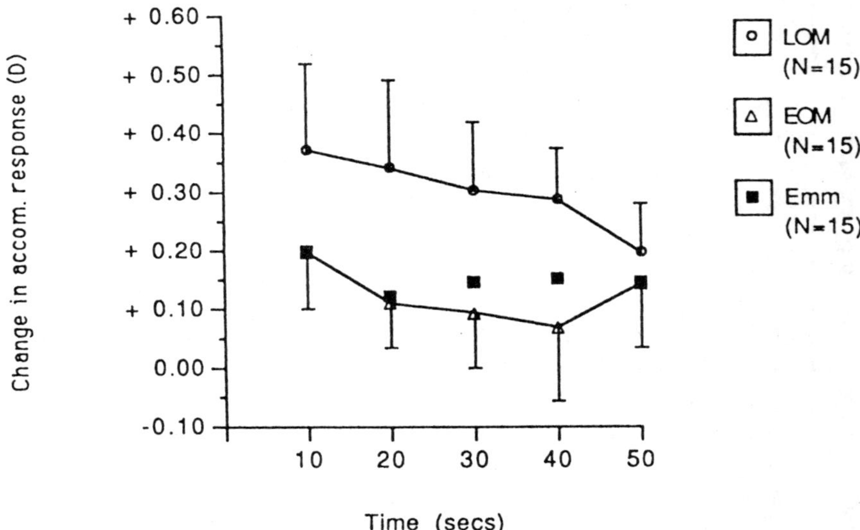

Figure 2-4 : Mean values of disparity-induced accommodation at the 2.50D accommodative stimulus level, the disparity being induced by the introduction of a 4pd base-out prism. LOM, late-onset myope; EOM, early-onset myope; Emm, emmetrope. Error bars indicate ± 1 SEM. Error bars have been omitted from the emmetropic data for clarity, but SEM's were of the order of ±0.09 (Reprinted with permission, Rosenfield and Gilmartin 1987c).

to an increased CA/C ratio, although the results of their later study (1988b) were not consistent with this idea (see preceding section). Alternatively, they also postulated that it might reflect an inability to relax blur-induced accommodation, which in turn was related to reduced sympathetic inhibitory innervation. In fact, the same study showed that late-onset myopes exhibited increased blur-induced accommodation. It thus appears that the latter hypothesis is more likely to be true, particularly in light of the fact that it is consistent with their data on convergent accommodation.

The above idea was supported by one of their later studies (Rosenfield and Gilmartin, 1988c). Ten emmetropes and 10 late-onset myopes (onset ≥15 years of age) were instructed to perform a counting task binocularly at 3 D, while their accommodation was assessed periodically over a 10-minute period with a Canon R-1 objective autorefractor. Disparity was introduced by addition of 3 and 6 p.d. base-out prism (total). Changes in the disparity stimulus did not result in any significant differences in the overall accommodative responses of the emmetropes, while the late-onset myopes exhibited significantly increased accommodative responses with increased disparity. Initial (t = 1 minute) values of disparity-induced accommodation were 0.10D and 0.13D for emmetropes and 0.25D and 0.34D for late-onset myopes for disparity stimuli of 3 and 6 p.d., respectively. Based on this result, the authors concluded that late-onset myopes exhibited higher levels of disparity-induced accommodation than emmetropes. However, further data analyses revealed that the significant difference between refractive groups occurred only for the accommodative response at the 0 prism or habitual congruent near condition (2.92D for emmetropes vs. 2.68D for late-onset myopes). It appears that the increase in disparity-induced accommodation in late-onset myopes effectively served to increase the overall accommodation level within the normal range to compensate for the initially low accommodative response for the 0 prism, the latter of which may be due to reduced myopic blur sensitivity (Gwiazda et al. 1993). It does not necessarily mean that late-onset myopes possess an increased responsivity to disparity stimulation per se as suggested earlier by these authors (1987c). Since measurements were obtained under closed-loop conditions, the contribution of blur accommodation and its interactions with disparity-induced accommodation must be taken into account. The authors further indicated that a greater proportion of disparity-induced accommodation might be involved in the normal accommodative response of the late-onset myopes versus the emmetropes. Since the aggregate accommodative response exhibited an increase, blur-induced accommodation must have either remained unchanged or increased, although the former seems more likely. The lack of change in blur accommodation could be attributed to the small magnitude of prisms used. As a consequence, the resultant changes in disparity-induced accommodation may not be sufficiently great to exceed the depth-of-focus, so that no compensatory response from blur accommodation was manifested. The lack of decrease in blur accommodation might also suggest an inability to reduce its response or an insensitivity to blur, which in turn might also explain the reduced response at 0 prism.

Alternatively, the data could be interpreted as reflecting decreased rather than increased disparity-induced accommodation in late-onset myopes; the reduced accommodative response found in late-onset myopes for a target at 3D without added prism might indicate a reduced input from disparity. Theoretically, with the introduction of an increased disparity stimulus, disparity-induced accommodation would be expected to increase with a concurrent attenuation of the blur accommodative component to maintain relative constancy of the steady-state accommodative response level. This was indeed reported for the emmetropes, so that accommodative responses for the 0, 3, and 6 p.d. conditions were statistically similar. In the late-onset myopes, however, blur accommodation must have failed to decrease to some extent, since the aggregate response increased relative to the habitual no-prism condition. The resultant increased accommodative response for either prism conditions was not significantly different when compared with the emmetropes. This might suggest that disparity-induced accommodation in late-onset myopes was initially reduced relative to the emmetropes under normal viewing conditions. Clearly, work in this area needs to be repeated in these populations under both open and closed-loop accommodative conditions with greater degrees of non-congruence for consistent and interpretable results to be found.

The more relevant question therefore is whether or not disparity-induced accommodation plays a role in the etiology of late-onset myopia. The authors suggested that the myopic onset may actually be an adaptive process, with its primary goal being the restoration of normal accommodation and vergence synkinesis. According to the nearpoint stress model postulated by Skeffington, such myopia must not be viewed as a problem but rather as an adaptive phenomenon secondary to near point stress-induced overconvergence. As a consequence, it serves to reduce accommodative demand and its associated accommodative convergence drive at the nearpoint (Birnbaum 1985).

Accommodative Vergence and the AC/A Ratio

Under normal binocular viewing conditions, a change in accommodation results in a binocularly-coordinated, concurrent change in vergence due to the synkinesis between the two systems (Ciuffreda and Kenyon 1983, Ciuffreda 1991, in press). This change in vergence is called accommodative vergence. The amount of change in accommodative vergence per unit change in accommodation is known as the response accommodative vergence to accommodation ratio, or the response AC/A ratio (Alpern and Larson 1960, Morgan 1968b). When the accommodative response is not measured but is assumed to equal the accommodative stimulus, then this is the stimulus AC/A ratio. The mean population clinical stimulus AC/A was found to be 4:1 (Morgan 1944, 1968a), with the response AC/A ratio being approximately 10% greater (Alpern et al. 1959).

Table 2-5 summarizes the findings and details pertinent to the studies on AC/A and refractive status. While Baldwin (1965) reported the absence of differences between his population of 80 early-onset myopes and that of the general population, the majority of studies have demonstrated otherwise. However, comparing Baldwin's data to that obtained for the general population is not representative of a veridical comparison for obvious reasons. For one, the general population data were derived from other studies, and methodological inconsistences are likely. Moreover, there is a strong possibility that the general subject population consisted of myopes as well, and this may have influenced the results in the direction of finding no difference. Subgroup refractive comparisons would best bring out such differences.

TABLE 2-5: SUMMARY RESULTS OF ACCOMMODATIVE VERGENCE AS A FUNCTION OF REFRACTIVE GROUP

INVESTIGATOR (YEAR)	DIAGNOSTIC CATEGORIES	N	AGES (yrs.)	APPARATUS	TARGET/DISTANCE	RESULTS
Manas (1955)	M (≥-2 sph) H (≥ +2 sph)	200	non-pres-byopes	subjective	6m & 40cm	M>H
Rosenfield & Gilmartin (1987a)	E (± 0.50 sph & ≤0.50 cyl) EOM (>-0.50 sph &<15y onset) LOM (-0.50 sph & ≥15y onset)	51	~21	infrared optometer & Maddox rod	N6 numbers @ 33cm & 3.9 & 4.6D	EOM>LOM=E
Jones (1990)	E (+0.75 to -0.25 sph) M (-1.25 to -3.50 sph)	48	N.A.	objective infrared systems	0 to 3D	M>E
Jiang (1995)	E (+0.37 to -0.25sph eq) LOM (≥ -0.37 sph eq) pre & post-onset (E who developed myopia >-0.50sph eq)	44	18-27	infrared optometer & dissociated phoria method	20/100 Snellen letters @ 2, .8 & .5m	LOM, pre-onset >E

In a study by Manas (1955), the clinical stimulus AC/A ratio was investigated as a function of refractive status. The AC/A was calculated from phoria measurements in a large population (n =200) consisting of non-presbyopic myopes and hyperopes. The AC/A (mean ± 1SD) for myopes (5.1± 2.1D) was significantly greater than that for hyperopes (4 ± 2.2 D). According to Manas, this difference in AC/A ratio was due to the fact that ametropes typically used "unequal" amounts of accommodation and convergence, with the myopes using considerably less accommodation than convergence, which eventually developed into an increased AC/A. Conversely, hyperopes characteristically used greater amounts of accommodation than convergence, thus resulting in a reduced AC/A. Unfortunately, no evidence was presented in support of these unusual ideas.

Manas' statement that myopes used substantially less accommodation than convergence may have been based on his presumption that ametropes habitually function with uncorrected vision. Such an ill-conceived notion precludes further discussion. In the case of corrected ametropia, however, several studies have previously reported that in general myopes exhibited reduced accommodation (Ramsdale 1979, McBrien and Millodot 1986b, Rosenfield and Gilmartin 1988c, Jones 1990, Bullimore et al. 1992, Gwiazda et al. 1993, 1995a), and this was in relation to other refractive groups and not relative to vergence. Admittedly, the reduced accommodation in myopes as noted in these studies was small, but it appeared to be of sufficient magnitude to account for the relatively small differences in the clinical stimulus AC/A ratios reported by Manas. Furthermore, the changes in direction of the AC/A ratios were not satisfactorily explained by Manas. It is known that for a unit of accommodation over the linear accommodative stimulus/response region (see Chapter 1), a constant amount of accommodative-vergence will be generated. Therefore, if myopes presumably accommodated less, then the response AC/A should remain constant *regardless* of the actual accommodation magnitude, while the stimulus AC/A should theoretically decrease and not increase as was reported by Manas. Moreover, the AC/A determined in this study was the stimulus AC/A and not the response AC/A, and therefore did not accurately reflect either true accommodation or the true AC/A ratio.

Despite the absence of a valid explanation, other studies have found similar results (Jones 1990). Response AC/A ratios were reported to be being significantly higher in myopes than in emmetropes. In an attempt to determine whether the etiology of late-onset myopia was related to the action of accommodation, vergence, or their mutual interactions, Rosenfield and Gilmartin (1987a) studied the response AC/A ratio in three refractive groups, namely emmetropia, early-onset myopia and late-onset myopia. The accommodative stimulus was positioned at 33cm. Negative spherical lenses were added to produce additional accommodative stimulus levels of 3.9 and 4.6D. To ensure accurate accommodation, subjects were required to perform a counting task during the measurements, and thus their attention and cognitive load were enhanced in addition to assuring actual resolution of the small targets. Steady-state accommodation was assessed objectively using the Canon R-1 Autoref infrared optometer, and its associated accommodative convergence was assessed subjectively using the clinical Maddox rod technique. Their results showed overall higher mean response AC/A ratios as compared with other studies (Flom and Takahashi 1962, Breinin and Chin 1972), and, in fact, were all outside normal limits (Borish 1970), which makes one question their methodology and thus their results and conclusions. The response AC/A ratios were significantly higher for early-onset myopes (9.55) relative to the late-onset myopes (7.61) and emmetropes (7.69), while the measured accommodative convergence per se between late-onset myopes and emmetropes was not significantly different. To determine if the difference between early- and late-onset myopes was due to variations in the degree of myopia, further analysis was performed on these subgroups after equating their myopia. The results confirmed the presence of a significant difference in AC/A ratio between the two groups.

This difference in AC/A ratios was explained in terms of the parameters described in the static accommodation and vergence model of Hung and Semmlow (1980). According to Rosenfield and Gilmartin (1987a), while overall accommodation (Rosenfield and Gilmartin 1987a) as well as the accommodative stimulus/response function (McBrien and Millodot 1986b), were reported to be similar between both subgroups, the difference in accommodative vergence can therefore only be ascribed to the presence of an increased gain factor (higher accommodative controller gain) in early-onset myopes, with this increase presumably being compensated for by an equivalent reduction in convergent accommodation. However, this notion was proven to be false in a subsequent study (Rosenfield and Gilmartin 1988b). Therefore, it appears that the higher AC/A ratios reported for myopes may be due to an increased crosslink gain rather than an increased accommodative controller gain, but this issue remains unresolved. Clearly, more work is needed in this important area.

More recently, Jiang (1995) evaluated the accommodative and vergence characteristics of 44 young adult subjects over the course of two to three years. Response AC/A ratios were determined at 6-month intervals. The data were analyzed in accordance with the refractive condition of the subject both at the commencement and conclusion of the study. In other words, subjects were classified as either belonging to the emmetropic group (emmetropes whose spherical equivalent refractive error remained in the +0.37 to -0.25D range), late-onset myopic group (whose initial refractive error

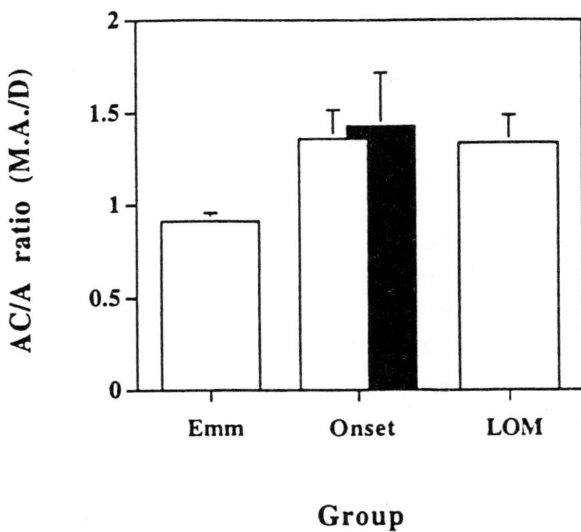

Figure 2-5 : AC/A ratio data averaged across subjects for the three groups. For the onset group's data, the open bar represents the mean of AC/A ratios of these subjects in the pre-onset period, and the filled bar represents the mean of AC/A ratios in the post-onset period. The error bars represent one standard error of the mean (Reprinted with permission, Jiang 1995).

exceeded -0.37D and continued to progress during the experiment) and onset group (emmetropes who developed myopia >-0.50D during the course of the study). The latter group was further subdivided into a pre-onset (when the refractive error remained <-0.50D) and a post-onset group (when the refractive error became ≥ -0.50D). Accommodation was measured objectively with an infrared optometer, while accommodative convergence was assessed subjectively using the flashed clinical dissociated phoria method. Mean response AC/A ratio (in units of meter angles per diopter and not prism diopters per diopter) for emmetropes (0.9) was significantly lower than the pre-onset and late-onset myopic group (~1.3), i.e., 5.4Δ/D versus 7.8Δ/D (Figure 2-5). It was also noted that the response AC/A increased during the development of myopia. It was further suggested that a high response AC/A ratio was a risk factor for myopic development. Assuming constancy of vergence, accommodation to near targets leads to increased accommodative lag in subjects with increased AC/A as compared to other subjects with normal or low AC/A. This accommodative lag results in increased defocus and/or blur, which may then act as an error signal for the growth mechanism of the eye, thus leading to axial myopia (See Chapter 6 on retinal defocus effects on myopic development).

From the foregoing, it appears that the response AC/A ratio does vary as a function of refractive status with it being highest in myopes, although the precise mechanism remains unclear. Further work is warranted.

Proximal Accommodation

It has been demonstrated that non-retinal factors can influence the state of accommodation (Ciuffreda 1991). One such factor is awareness of the perceived or apparent target distance as well as one's overall surround or propinquity (Rosenfield and Ciuffreda 1991). The accommodation derived as a consequence of this near perceptual awareness is most aptly termed proximal accommodation. Perceived target nearness can be changed by either direct means, i.e., altering the physical distance of a target in free space, or by indirect means, i.e., by altering target size (in a cue-free environment) and thereby altering its perceived distance (Grant 1942). Previous studies have employed both techniques under either single or double open- and closed-loop conditions and have reported mixed results (Ittleson and Ames 1950, Alpern 1958, Morgan 1962, Hennessy and Leibowitz 1971, Kruger and Pola 1985, Rosenfield and Gilmartin 1990, Rosenfield and Ciuffreda 1991, Rosenfield et al. 1991).

Under open-loop conditions, i.e., when both the blur-driven accommodative and disparity vergence inputs were eliminated, proximal accommodation has been shown to have a substantial motor contribution. In a study by Rosenfield and Gilmartin (1990), in which the actual target distance in physical space was either 33cm or 5m while its angular subtense remained constant, a proximal gain of approximately 0.6 was found. That is, for every 1D change in target distance, accommodation changed by 0.6D. A later study (Rosenfield et al. 1991), in which the actual target distance ranged from 20 cm to 1500m, showed an overall gain of 0.45 with changes occurring in a linear manner from 20cm to 3m; from 3m and beyond, there was no proximal drive to accommodation. These open-loop values are consistent with a mathematical analysis performed by Hung et al. (1996) based on a comprehensive static accommodative and vergence model. The results of these studies clearly demonstrate that under open-loop conditions, the oculomotor response is clearly driven by perceived distance. Similarly, the proximally-induced effect can even be demonstrated in the *absence* of a visible target. For example, tonic accommodation was significantly altered when subjects had full knowledge of test room dimensions and its overall topography, i.e., propinquity effect (Rosenfield and Ciuffreda 1991). Thus, since tonic accommodation per se is constant, the measurement difference was due to proximal accommodation.

Under naturalistic binocular closed-loop viewing conditions, however, the contribution of proximal accommodation to the overall steady-state accommodative level is very small. Based on the accommodation and vergence model parameters, the proximal input was calculated to be only about 4% (Hung et al. 1996). This is consistent with earlier empirical findings. Ittleson and Ames (1950), employing the approach of altering target size, found a small but consistent change in steady-state accommodation of 0.25-0.50D. In contrast, Alpern (1958) found no difference under similar conditions. More recent studies by Rosenfield et al. (1990) and Jones (1993), using the paradigm of altered physical distance, demonstrated that the within-task overall accommodative response for equidioptric targets placed at far and near distances showed no significant difference. In addition, in the former study (Rosenfield et al. 1990), the mean accommodative adaptation following the near versus far tasks was also equivalent. However, there was a significant positive correlation between the individual subject's level of adaptation at far versus near, indicating that the initial adaptation induced after the near viewing distance was approximately twice that found for the equidioptric distance adaptation task. These results suggest that the proximal drive to accommodation may actually be considerable, especially with respect to adaptive aspects, although this effect is not manifested nor can it be measured under naturalistic closed-loop conditions due to the dominance of blur and depth-of-focus constraints in the control of accommodation (Ciuffreda 1991, Hung et al. 1996).

TABLE 2-6: SUMMARY RESULTS OF PROXIMALLY-INDUCED ACCOMMODATION AS A FUNCTION OF REFRACTIVE GROUP

INVESTI-GATOR	DIAGNOSTI C CATEGORIES	N	AGES (yrs.)	APPAR-ATUS	TARGET/ DISTANCE	RESULTS
Rosenfield & Gilmartin (1990)	E (± 0.50 sph & ≤0.50 cyl) LOM (-1.00 to -3.25 sph, ≤1.00 cyl & ≥15y onset)	20	~23	Canon R-1 infrared optometer	6/6 letters @ 5m or 33 cm with 0.5mm monocular pinhole	E>LOM

Proximal accommodation has been shown to vary as a function of refractive state (Table 2-6). Rosenfield and Gilmartin (1990) studied emmetropes (n =10) and late-onset myopes (n =10). Targets were viewed monocularly through a 0.5mm pinhole, thus rendering both blur-driven accommodation and disparity vergence open-loop. The targets were placed at 5m and 0.33m, and accommodation was assessed objectively using a Canon R-1 Autoref infrared optometer. The difference in accommodative response between the two target distances represented proximally-driven accommodation. Significant increases in proximal accommodation, ranging from 0.80-1.70 D, were found when viewing the near versus far target. Moreover, proximal accommodation in the emmetropes was significantly greater than in the late-onset myopes (Figure 2-6). Initial mean proximal

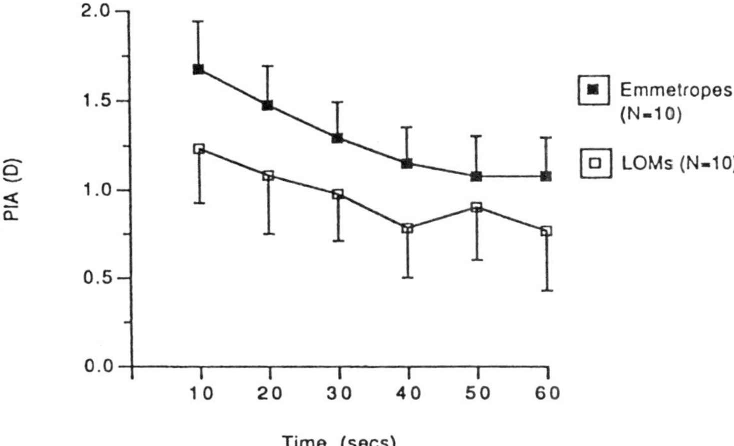

Figure 2-6 : Mean value of proximally-induced accommodation (PIA) for 10 emmetropes and 10 late-onset myopes during the course of a 60-s fixation period. PIA was calculated as the difference in open-loop accommodative response when viewing targets located at viewing distances of 0.2D and 3.0D. Error bars represent ± 1 SEM. (Reprinted with permission, Rosenfield and Gilmartin 1990).

accommodation of 1.70D and 1.25D, with a maximum gain (ratio of proximal accommodative response/accommodative stimulus) of 0.6 and 0.3, was observed for emmetropes and late-onset myopes, respectively. At first glance, this difference suggests a reduced perceptual or proximal gain. This is a strange conclusion, however, as it is not clear why having myopia, especially of relatively low magnitude, should change one's basic visual perception so dramatically. However, an alternative explanation that seems more plausible is that myopes simply have slightly lower accommodative gain, as they accommodate less than emmetropes for either blur only (Gwiazda et al. 1993) or in this case proximal only stimulation. Thus, at least theoretically, such reduced proximal accommodation in late-onset myopes would necessitate increased blur and vergence-driven accommodation under normal binocular near viewing conditions for some given level of accommodation at near. On the other hand, if proximal accommodation in late-onset myopes is reduced, and this difference is not compensated for by an increase in blur and/or vergence-driven accommodative components, a slightly decreased overall accommodative response would result. In fact, reduced accommodation in myopes appears to be the case (Gwiazda et al. 1993). If this reduction is considerable, it would suggest an increased depth-of-focus in late-onset myopes, so that the increased retinal defocus resulting from the larger accommodative lag would not be appreciated. However, although the proximal contribution under normal closed-loop

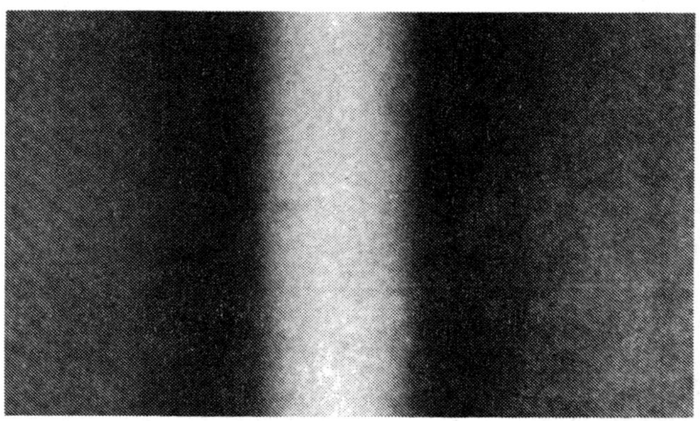

Figure 2-7 : Difference of gaussian target, more commonly referred to as DOG.

viewing conditions is minimal (Rosenfield et al. 1990, Hung et al. 1996), probably even in late-onset myopes, this proximal (perceptual) input would now act as a potent reinforcing stimulus in conjunction with the other sensory inputs to assist the accommodative motor system.

How might this relate to the etiology of myopia? Any increased defocus (subthreshold or otherwise) that occurs as a consequence of a reduced steady-state accommodative response might trigger the development of myopia (Held et al. 1994). This line of argument is supported predominantly by animal studies in which either defocus or visual deprivation during the critical developmental period has led to myopia (Wiesel and Raviola 1977, Wallman 1987, Ni and Smith 1989), and in human studies where eyes deprived of adequate visual stimulation, such as occurs with corneal and lenticular opacities, developed high degrees of myopia (Rabin 1981, Johnson et al. 1982). See Chapters 4, 6 and 7 for further discussions.

Tonic Accommodation

Tonic accommodation is defined as the response of the accommodative system in the absence of visual stimuli, such as blur, disparity and proximity (Rosenfield et al. 1993). It is measured under one of the following conditions: in total darkness, in a contrastless field or "ganzfeld," or under open-loop conditions, e.g., with a clinical difference-of-gaussian target (Wesson and Koenig 1983, Kotulak and Schor 1987) (Figure 2-7) or when viewing through a pinhole monocularly. Under the aforementioned conditions, there is a lack of an adequate visual stimulus to accommodation. In other words, there is an absence of stimuli changes concurrent with the accommodative changes, so that the quality of the retinal image is independent of the eye's state of focus. The accommodative response, devoid of inputs from the different accommodative components, assumes a mean baseline level of approximately 0.5-1.0D as measured with an open-field infrared optometer in a large room (Rosenfield et al. 1993). It remains stable over an extended period of time (Owens and Higgins 1983). Various terms such as dark focus, dark accommodation, resting point of accommodation, and abias have been used as synonyms for tonic accommodation.

Studies investigating the relationship between tonic accommodation and ocular refraction have resulted in conflicting results. A majority of them showed that hyperopes exhibited the highest tonic accommodation followed by emmetropes and then myopes (Table 2-7a) (Irving 1957, Maddock et al. 1981, Smith 1983, Heron et al. 1984, McBrien and Millodot 1987, Bullimore and Gilmartin 1987, Rosenfield and Gilmartin 1987, Bullimore et al. 1988, McBrien and Millodot 1988, Gilmartin et al. 1989a, Rosner and Rosner 1989, Gilmartin and Bullimore 1991, Hung and Ciuffreda 1991, Rosenfield and Ciuffreda 1991, Miwa 1992, Adams and McBrien 1993, Miwa and Tokoro 1993a, b, Gwiazda et al. 1995b, Jiang 1995), while a few studies found the opposite (Table 2-7b) (Suzumura 1979, Gawron 1981, Simonelli 1983). Several other studies, however, showed no significant difference between refractive subgroups (Table 2-7c) (Carreras 1951, Braddick et al. 1981, Maddock et al. 1981, Ramsdale 1985, Fisher et al. 1987, Bullimore and Gilmartin 1987, Rosenfield and Gilmartin 1988a, Rosenfield and Gilmartin 1989, Rosenfield and Gilmartin 1990, Gilmartin and Bullimore 1991, Morse and Smith 1993, Woung et al. 1993, Strang et al. 1994). It appears that these differences between studies may be attributed, but not limited, to one or a combination of the following factors: mode of measurement/instrumentation, viewing condition, cognitive demand, subject population, and refractive error criterion. In conditions other than darkness, e.g., when either a degraded or an open-loop visual stimulus were present, or when measurement of tonic accommodation was subjective, i.e., the subject actively participated and consciously exerted effort to judge the direction of the optometer target movement as in the laser or Hartinger coincidence optometers, tonic accommodative values were comparatively higher in contrast to those obtained objectively with an infrared optometer (Post et al. 1984, 1985, Rosenfield 1989). In either case, although the optometer targets were open-loop and therefore should not constitute a good blur-driven accommodative stimulus, the presence of an isolated open-loop visual target allowed proximal and/or cognitive influences to manifest themselves, resulting in inflated tonic accommodation values (Rosenfield and Gilmartin 1990, Rosenfield and Ciuffreda 1990, Winn et al. 1991). In addition, even when using a similar type of instrumentation, tonic accommodation has been found to vary with the amount of mental effort invoked, with this effect varying across refractive groups (Jaschinski-Kruza and Toenies 1988, Winn et al. 1991).

For example, Bullimore and Gilmartin (1987) found that different values were obtained for passive versus active conditions, with the latter yielding

TABLE 2-7a: SUMMARY RESULTS OF TONIC ACCOMMODATION AS A FUNCTION OF REFRACTIVE GROUP

INVESTIGATOR (YEAR)	DIAGNOSTIC CATEGORIES	N	AGES (yrs.)	APPARATUS	CONDITION	RESULTS
Irving (1957)	E M H	50	N.A.	Ruka Variator	low luminance (0.02cd/m^2)	H>E, M
Maddock, Millodot, Leat & Johnson (Davis) (1981)	E (plano) low M(<-3sph) highM(>-3sph)	40	<25	laser optometer	N.A.	E>high M
Smith (1983)	E (+2.25 to -1.25 sph) H (≤+2.25 sph) M (≤-1.25 sph)	13	19-43	laser optometer	darkness, empty field	H>M (weak r= -0.49, p =0.10)
Heron, Bahri, Burnside, Kacouli , Mackintosh (1984)	E (±3 sph) M (>-3sph) H (>+3 sph)	57	N.A.	laser optometer	N.A.	H>M
McBrien & Millodot (1987)	E (range -0.25 to +0.75 sph eq & ≤1cyl) H (>+0.75 sph eq & ≤1cyl) EM (>-0.25 sph eq, ≤1cyl &13y onset) LOM >(-0.25 sph eq, ≤1cyl &≤15y onset)	62	19-25	infrared optometer	darkness	H>E=EOM>LOM
Bullimore & Gilmartin (Passive) (1987)	E (plano to +0.50 sph & ≤0.50 cyl) LOM (-0.50 to -3.50 sph, ≤0.50 cyl & ≥15y onset)	30	19-26	infrared optometer	darkness	E>LOM (trend)
Rosenfield & Gilmartin (1987a)	E (± 0.50 sph & ≤0.50 cyl) EOM (>-0.50 sph &<15 y onset) LOM (>-0.50 sph & ≤15y onset)	51	~21	infrared optometer	darkness	E>LOM E=EOM EOM=LOM

Bullimore, Boyd, Mather, Gilmartin (1988)	E LOM EOM H	100	18-29	retinoscope	N.A.	H>E>LOM,EOM
McBrien & Millodot (1988)	E (+0.75 to -0.25 sph eq) H (>+0.75 sph eq) EOM (>-0.25 sph eq&≤13y) LOM >-0.25 sph eq&≤15y)	47	18-27	infrared optometer	darkness	H>E,EOM>LOM
Gilmartin, Bullimore, Rosenfield & Winn (1989)	E LOM	30	N.A.	infrared optometer	darkness	E>LOM
Rosner & Rosner (1989)	E (+0.75 to -0.25 sph) M (>-0.25sph) H (>+0.75 sph)	113	6-14	retinoscope	0.2cpd dim difference-of-gaussian @ 40 cm	H>E>M
Gilmartin & Bullimore (1991)	E (plano to +0.50 sph eq &≤ 0.50cyl) LOM (-0.50 to -2.25 sph eq & ≤0.50 cyl & >15y)	30	19-25	infrared optometer	darkness	@ 1 & 5D: E>LOM
Hung & Ciuffreda (1991)	E (± 0.75sph) low M (-0.75 to -4 sph) highM (-4sph) H (>+0.75sph)	48	21-35	Hartinger coincidence optometer	darkness	high M= E> low M, H
Rosenfield & Ciuffreda (1991)	E (± 0.50 sph & ≤0.50 cyl) M ($\bar{x}$= -3.12 sph eq & ≤1 cyl)	10	22-36	infrared optometer	darkness	E>M
Miwa (1992)	+8 to -11 sph	105	4-20	infrared optometer	darkness	low H>M,highH

Adams & McBrien (1993)	E LOM	164	21-55	infrared optometer	darkness	E>M
Miwa & Tokoro (1993a)	<-2 sph >-2 sph	19	19-20	infrared optometer	darkness	low M> high M
Miwa & Tokoro (1993b)	mean= +0.32sph	196	4-17	infrared optometer	darkness	H>M
Gwiazda, Bauer, Thorn, Held (1995b)	E (+0.75 to -0.25 sph) M (-0.25 to -7.00 sph eq) H (+1 to +4.12 sph)	87	6.5-16.5	infrared optometer	darkness	H,E>M
Jiang (1995)	E (+0.37 to -0.25 sph eq) LOM (≥-0.37 sph eq) pre & post-≥onset (E who developed myopia > -0.50 sph eq)	44	18-27	infrared optometer	darkness	pre-onset>E>LOM

TABLE 2-7b: SUMMARY RESULTS OF TONIC ACCOMMODATION AS A FUNCTION OF REFRACTIVE GROUP

INVESTIGATOR (YEAR)	DIAGNOSTIC CATEGORIES	N	AGES (yrs.)	APPARATUS	CONDITIO N	RESULTS
Suzumura (1979)	E M H	126	5-49	infrared optometer	N.A.	mild M(1-3 sph) >E, advanced M
Gawron (1981)	E (pl to -1 sph) M (> -1 sph) H (≥+0.25 sph)	152	17-28	polarized vernier optometer	N.A.	M>H>E
Simonelli (1983)	E, M, H (+4.5 to -12.6 sph)	301	16-67	N.A.	N.A.	M>E >H

TABLE 2-7c: SUMMARY RESULTS OF TONIC ACCOMMODATION AS A FUNCTION OF REFRACTIVE GROUP

INVESTIGATOR (YEAR)	DIAGNOSTIC CATEGORIES	N	AGES (yrs.)	APPARATUS	CONDITION	RESULTS
Carreras (1951)	E (<± 2 sph) H (+2 to +5 sph) M (-4 to -21 sph)	21	N.A.	N.A.	minimum light threshold for detection of distant Landolt C gap	E=H=M
Braddick, Ayling, Sawyer & Atkinson (1981)	E (± 0.25 sph) H (<+4.50 sph) M (<.50 sph)	23	18-34	photo-refraction	darkness	E=H=M
Maddock, Millodot, Leat & Johnson (Cardiff) (1981)	E (± 2 sph) H (<+2 to +4 sph) M (-2 to -7 sph)	23	<25	laser optometer	darkness	E=H=M
Ramsdale (1985)	E (± -0.50 sph & <1cyl) H (+0.50 to +5.50 sph & <1cyl) LOM (-0.50 to -7.75 sph & <1cyl)	40	18-34	laser optometer	Snellen (6/ 3-6/1 9)	E=H= M TA=intercept
Fisher, Ciuffreda & Levine (1987)	E (± 0.75) H (>+0.75sph) low M (>-0.75 but ≤-4 sph) highM(>-4sph)	48	21-35	Hartinger optometer	open-loop optometer target in darkness	E=H=low M=high M
Bullimore & Gilmartin (Active) (1987)	E (plano to +0.50 sph & ≤0.50 cyl) LOM (-0.50 to –3.50 sph, ≤0.50 cyl & ≥5y onset)	30	19-26	infrared optometer	darkness with cognitive task	E=LOM
Rosenfield & Gilmartin (1988a)	E (± 0.50 sph & ≤ 0.50 cyl) LOM (-0.75 to -4 sph & ≥15y onset)	20	~22	infrared optometer	darkness	E=LOM

Rosenfield & Gilmartin (1989)	E (± 0.50 sph & ≤ 0.50 cyl) LOM (>-0.50 sph, ≤1cyl & ≥15y onset)	20	~22	infrared optometer	darkness	E=LOM
Rosenfield & Gilmartin (1990)	E (± 0.50 sph & ≤0.50 cyl) LOM (-1.00 to -3.25 sph, ≤ 1.00 cyl & ≥15y onset)	20	~23	infrared optometer	darkness	E=LOM
Gilmartin & Bullimore (1991)	E (plano to +0.50 sph eq & ≤0.50 cyl) LOM (-0.50 to -2.25 sph eq & ≤ 0.50 cyl & >15y)	30	19-25	infrared optometer	darkness	@ 3D:E=LOM
Morse & Smith (1993)	E (+0.75 to -0.50 sph) EOM (>-0.50 sph & <14y onset) LOM (> -0.50 sph & >15y onset)	28	22-30	infrared optometer and eyetracker	N.A.	E=EOM=LOM
Woung, Ukai, Tsuchiya & Ishikawa (1993)	E (+0.75 to -0.25 sph) EOM (> -0.50 sph & ≤1cyl & ≤13y) LOM (> -0.50 sph & ≤1cyl & ≥15y)	51	19-38	infrared optometer	internal asterisk @ 8D	E=LOM=EOM
Strang, Winn & Gilmartin (1994)	E (+0.50 to -0.25 sph & ≤0.50 cyl) LOM(-1.00 to -3.25 sph & ≤0.50 cyl & >15y onset)	20	~23	infrared optometer	darkness	E=LOM

higher values. Thirty age-matched emmetropes and late-onset myopes were tested. Tonic accommodation was assessed objectively with the Canon R-1 infrared optometer while the subject sat in darkness under 2 conditions: (1) the passive condition which involved minimal mental effort, and (2) the active condition which required subjects to perform reverse counting which involved greater mental effort. Under the former condition, a trend was demonstrated with emmetropes exhibiting slightly higher tonic accommodation (1.14D) relative to the late-onset myopes (0.81D). On the other hand, no significant difference was found between refractive groups for the active condition; i.e., 1.21D versus 1.16D for the emmetropes and the late-onset myopes, respectively, presumably due to increased variability. For both groups, the active condition was found to induce higher tonic values. This cognitively-induced shift for late-onset myopes (0.35D) was significantly greater than for the emmetropes (0.07). It is not known if this susceptibility for differential component innervation between refractive groups transfers to other accommodative demand tasks. Therefore, to make an appropriate comparison of tonic accommodation between refractive subgroups, it is essential that extraneous factors such as proximity and cognitive factors be eliminated or at the least be held constant across all subgroups. This becomes critical as these parameters have been demonstrated to exert a differential effect in the various refractive subgroups (Rosenfield and Gilmartin 1990, Bullimore et al. 1992).

A similar situation was found in a study by Rosner and Rosner (1989). Using an entirely different experimental paradigm and instrumentation, tonic accommodation of 6 to 14-year-old children was assessed. The subjects fixated upon a dimly lit and blur-free 0.2cpd clinical difference-of-gaussian target (Wesson and Koenig 1983) positioned at 40 cm, while their accommodation was measured via dynamic retinoscopy. The results revealed that tonic accommodation in hyperopes was significantly greater than the emmetropes and myopes. Although the target used was in the open-loop mode, nonetheless, positioning it at a near distance may pose a problem. It may have introduced proximal cues which, in all likelihood, would have contaminated and elevated the tonic accommodation measures. In fact, several investigations showed that when measuring accommodation under dual open-loop conditions, which theoretically should yield "pure" tonic accommodation values, significant increases in the measured response were observed following repositioning of the target from a range of far to near distances or when the subject was cognizant of surround propinquity (Rosenfield and Gilmartin 1990, Rosenfield and Ciuffreda 1991, Rosenfield et al. 1991). This demonstrated the potent effect of the awareness of a proximal stimulus on tonic accommodation, especially in this dual open-loop mode (Hung et al. 1996). No significant difference in tonic accommo-

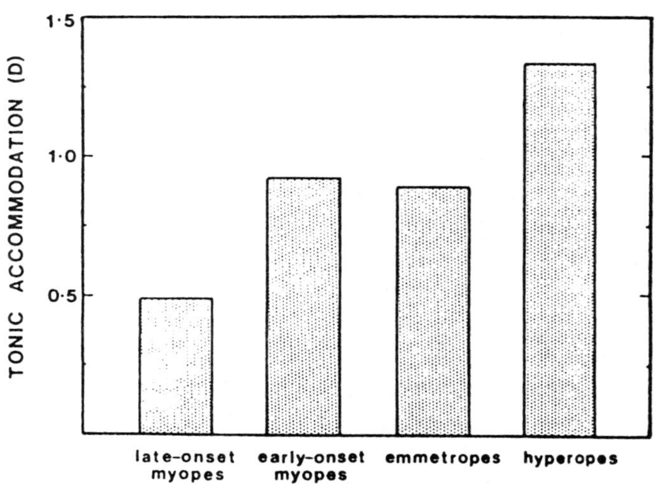

Figure 2-8 : Differences in the mean dioptric value of tonic accommodation for 15 corrected late-onset myopes, 15 corrected early-onset myopes, 17 emmetropes, and 15 corrected hyperopes (Reprinted with permission, McBrien and Millodot 1987).

dation was found between emmetropes and late-onset myopes under the far target condition; however, a significant difference was noted when the target was placed at near, as mentioned earlier.

In addition to the above, other factors may account for some of the differences between studies. Firstly, there is the refractive criterion. Maddock et al. (1981) reported conflicting data for populations from different geographic locations (Cardiff and Davis). This can probably be attributed to differences in their refractive criterion. The refractive category for emmetropes in the Cardiff population covered a relatively wide refractive range (± 2D from true emmetropia). Thus, some low ametropes were likely to be included in the sample. Secondly, when the subject population consisted of young children, Miwa and Tokoro (1993b) demonstrated that the relation between refractive groups was dependent on effective cycloplegia. In the absence of cycloplegia, tonic accommodation was not found to vary with refraction. However, when cycloplegic refraction was used as the reference baseline, hyperopic eyes showed greater tonic accommodation values than emmetropes, which was similar to the Rosner and Rosner (1989) non-cycloplegic DOG results.. Finally, equating the tonic accommodation value with the intercept of the accommodative stimulus/response function and the unit ratio line, as was done by Ramsdale (1985), has been demonstrated to be inaccurate and not representative of the veridical tonic accommodation value (Rosenfield et al. 1993).

A comparative study was conducted between all refractive groups (emmetropes, hyperopes, early and late-onset myopes) (McBrien and Millodot

1987). The results revealed significant differences between all possible pairs except between the emmetropes and early-onset myopes, with hyperopes exhibiting the greatest amount of tonic accommodation and late-onset myopes the least (Figure 2-8). However, the correlation between refractive group and tonic accommodation was low (r = +0.24), suggesting a weak relationship. Nonetheless, in consideration of the possibility of a differential tonic accommodation value across refractive groups, what could be the explanation and its implications? The authors discussed interpretations of their findings based on the theories of autonomic innervation proposed by different investigators (Charman 1982, Garner 1983). These theories were primarily based on Toates' model of accommodation (Toates 1970, 1972) and related tonic accommodation and refractive error to the relative contribution of the parasympathetic and sympathetic branches of the autonomic nervous systems.

The main objections to these ideas as well as to Toates' model itself include the following:

1) they postulated that upon full correction of myopia, all points on the accommodative stimulus/response function including tonic accommodation were shifted to lower dioptric values. This should indeed be true, as now the uncorrected refractive bias is removed. However, the dioptric difference between the far point and tonic accommodation should remain unchanged. Therefore, the recorded value may change dioptrically but the tonic accommodative value per se has not changed;
2) as mentioned earlier, however, equating the intersection of the accommodative stimulus/response function with the 1:1 demand line to the tonic accommodation level was erroneous (Rosenfield et al. 1993).
3) tonic accommodation was assumed to be at and represent the equilibrium position between the parasympathetic and sympathetic innervations. Distant accommodation, i.e., accommodation to targets farther than this cross-over position presumed to represent tonic accommodation would be accomplished by sympathetic innervation and, conversely, parasympathetic innervation would be used for near accommodation. However, as was addressed in McBrien and Millodot (1987), this notion has been disproved by Tornqvist (1967). Moreover, other work suggested that variations in tonic accommodation were a consequence of variations in parasympathetic tone of the ciliary muscle (Gilmartin and Hogan 1985a).

The most plausible interpretation of their results was that myopes exhibited an overall reduced autonomic innervation. More importantly, they related their findings of reduced tonic accommodation to research results pertaining to accommodative hysteresis, with the two being characterized by an inverse relation (Ebenholtz 1985). Thus, one would predict greater myopic or inward shifts in the myopes (Ebenholtz 1985, Morse and Smith 1993). In addition, since sympathetic innervation is inhibitory in nature, and its proposed function is attenuation of post-task myopic shifts, a reduced sympathetic facility would indeed result in greater shifts. This could have important implications in theories of refractive development, and it will be discussed in subsequent chapters.

The majority of results suggests reduced tonic accommodation in late-onset myopes, although there are notable exceptions. Thus, the relationship is weak at best. One possible reason for this may lie in the experimental methodology which lent itself to contamination by other extraneous inputs, e.g., proximal and cognitive influences, as discussed previously. In an attempt to summarize the various findings, Fisher et al. (1987) combined data obtained across several studies including their own which used different types of instrumentation. A complex curvilinear relation between tonic accommodation and refractive error was indicated. Tonic accommodation appeared to be least for low myopia (1-5D) and increased slightly for higher myopia and hyperopia. However, the significance of these findings is still unclear. Control system modelling has indicated that the tonic contribution to the aggregate accommodative response under normal closed-loop viewing conditions is minimal (Hung and Semmlow 1980). Therefore, its impact under naturalistic viewing conditions appears not to be great, and hence it would not be expected to play a significant role in myopia as related to accommodative responsivity per se.

To investigate the relation between tonic accommodation and the development of myopia, two longitudinal studies have been conducted. Owens et al. (1989) examined a small sample of high school and college students. Unfortunately, the results were equivocal. Although parallel time-related changes in tonic accommodation and myopic refractive development were demonstrated for the group data, these measures were not strongly correlated for the individual subjects. However, lower tonic accommodation appeared to be related to an increased rate of myopic progression. In the second study, Jiang (1995) demonstrated that the magnitude of tonic accommodation may be related to the time of onset of myopia. For example, Jiang (1995) showed that late onset myopes exhibited significantly reduced tonic accommodation relative to emmetropes. However, emmetropes who were in the process of developing myopia displayed significantly elevated tonic accommodation prior to myopic onset, which gradually lowered following its onset. Reduced tonic accommodation was manifested only after the subjects became myopic for a period of time. Thus, refractive group differences in tonic accommodation may depend on when tonic accommodation is measured. Accordingly, it was suggested that a high level of tonic accommodation may be a risk factor for the development of myopia in an emmetrope.

A few notable investigators also placed importance on the role of tonic accommodation and implicated it as the antecedent of myopia. For example, Van Alphen (1961) proposed that the refractive state was determined by the "stretch" factor, and that myopization or the amount of stretch was regulated by the resistance offered by the choroid and ciliary muscle which behaved as a continuous coat and functioned as a single unit. The potential to stretch due to increased intraocular pressure would be counteracted by choroidal tension, which in turn was related to the tonus of the ciliary muscle. Therefore, high ciliary muscle tone would be predicted to offer increased resistance to stretching, and conversely low ciliary muscle tone (or low tonic accommodation) would be predicted to offer decreased resistance to stretching and therefore predispose one to axial elongation and hence myopic development. By the same token, myopia resulting from axial elongation due theoretically to the inability to resist stretch must possess low tone and hence reduced tonic accommodation. (See Chapter 4 for a fuller discussion of this notion).

Accommodative Adaptation

Immediately following a sustained accommodative task, the remeasured "tonic accommodative level" will be biased in the direction of this immediately preceding task. This associated directional response bias or aftereffect is known as accommodative adaptation/hysteresis (Ebenholtz 1983, Schor et al. 1986). The accommodative system has been demonstrated to be quite susceptible to hysteresis effects, since significant adaptation has been reported to occur for periods of sustained near focus as brief as 15 seconds (Rosenfield and Gilmartin 1989, Fisher et al. 1990). The decay of the aftereffect was reported to last from several seconds (Gilmartin and Bullimore 1987, Gilmartin et al. 1989a) to a few minutes (Wolf et al. 1987), and perhaps even hours (Ebenholtz 1983). Thus, this relatively extended time course of accommodative decay was the premise that initially led some investigators to postulate an association between sustained nearwork and the development of myopia. See later discussion in this chapter and also Chapter 4.

One of the most oft-cited studies in this area was performed by Ebenholtz, who demonstrated the existence of accommodative hysteresis (Ebenholtz 1983) and further indicated that the magnitude of the shift was dependent upon the level of pre-task tonic accommodation (Ebenholtz 1985). In his initial study, Ebenholtz (1983) used a laser optometer to record the tonic accommodative level of 12 emmetropes prior to and following an 8-minute fixation task. The target was placed at the linear equivalent of the subject's near point, far point and tonic accommodative level. Significant mean myopic shifts of 0.34 D and hyperopic shifts of 0.21 D were evident for the majority of subjects following a near point fixation and far point fixation task, respectively. This inequality in shift magnitude was, according to the author, related to the departure of the dioptric equivalent of the stimulus from the pre-task tonic accommodative level. Therefore, for an equivalent accommodative task demand, one would predict greater myopic shifts for myopes, since they have been reported to have reduced tonic accommodative levels.

The temporal aspects of accommodative hysteresis were also investigated in the same study. The shifts appeared to be relatively long-lived. The decay in the dark was calculated to be completed in approximately 1 hour following the far task and 10 hours for near task based on the criterion of 5 time constants (Ebenholtz 1983). However, re-analysis of the data by Rosenfield et al. (1994) indicated that the post-task tonic accommodation following the near task was no longer statistically different from baseline in approximately 25-50 minutes, which is still quite long. Moreover, the laser optometer used in the study has inherent limitations, such that both a proximal (Rosenfield 1989) as well as a cognitive component (Post et al. 1984) were probably present, which would act to increase hysteresis magnitude and duration. Furthermore, much shorter decay times have been reported by other investigators using more optimal devices. For example, Wolf et al. (1987) demonstrated accommodative hysteresis which lasted for only 3 minutes following a 45-minute interrupted task as measured with the haploscope optometer using the principle of stigmatoscopy. Studies using the infra-red optometer demonstrated an even more rapid decline to baseline with post-task tonic accommodation recovering to baseline within 60 seconds (Gilmartin et al. 1989a). And, if one considers the fact that such accommodative-adaptive effects under naturalistic conditions occur not in darkness but rather in the presence of visual feedback, then this should act to cause such effects to dissipate even more rapidly. See chapter 4.

Comparative studies on accommodative hysteresis have revealed differences between various refractive groups (Table 2-8). McBrien and Millodot (1988) showed that late-onset myopes exhibited significantly greater accommodative adaptation than the other groups following a counting task performed at 20 cm for 15 minutes. Adaptation was not evident for their early-onset myopes and emmetropes, while hyperopes exhibited counteradaptive shifts. For tasks performed at a farther distance of 37cm, a similar pattern was demonstrated but with smaller magnitude shifts. Not surprisingly, at a task distance of 6m, no adaptation was reported for late-onset myopes, while hyperopic shifts were manifested by the remaining groups. In contrast to the other refractive groups, adaptation for late-onset myopes to all near tasks failed to decay fully within the 15-minute post-task monitoring period.

This trend was also evident for tasks of brief durations. Following a 2-minute task at 4D, accommodative adaptation was shown to vary as a function of refraction (Woung et al. 1993). Late-onset myopes had significantly greater adaptation (1.19D) relative to early-onset myopes (0.40D) throughout the entire duration of the 5-minute post-task measurement period and relative to the emmetropes (0.59D) for the time beyond 200s, while adaptation between emmetropes and early-onset myopes was significantly different only during the initial 3 minutes of the post-task period. When adaptation was analyzed in terms of age of myopic onset, no clear correlation was found. However, the largest shifts occurred for a myopic onset of approximately 15 years of age, which would therefore be found in late-onset myopes. This may be a factor in late-onset myopia, and it deserves further investigation.

Refractive group differences may also relate to variations in task duration and dioptric demand. While presence of accommodative hysteresis appeared to be somewhat independent of ocular refraction, differences in magnitude and temporal characteristics of this accommodative adaptation between refractive groups have been shown to vary with task duration (Rosenfield and Gilmartin 1989). Although no significant differences between emmetropes and late-onset myopes were found for either the 15 or 30-second task, the longer task duration of 45s revealed a modified regression pattern for late-onset myopes. Negative (i.e., counteradaptive) post-task shifts were manifested. These shifts were presumed to be mediated via adrenergic innervation, since they could be abolished with the instillation of timolol maleate (Figure 2-9). Additional evidence was provided by its time of onset which also lent support to the work of Tornqvist (1967), who demonstrated that sympathetic stimulation developed slowly reaching a maximum after 10-40 seconds. Thus, only with relatively long periods of continuous focus could the sympathetic system potentially influence accommodation and the far point of the eye.

Adaptation differences also appeared to be influenced by the accommodative demand. Gilmartin and Bullimore (1991) studied adaptation and its decay in emmetropes and late-onset myopes using tasks whose dioptric demands were equivalent to 1, 3 and 5D. Interestingly, significant refractive group differences in adaptation magnitude were only reported for the 1D task, with late-onset myopes having greater shifts than emmetropes. Its decay was faster for emmetropes than late-onset myopes for the 3 and 5D tasks. These decay differences cannot be attributed to variations in within-task accommodation or tonic accommodation, since the recorded responses between groups were either equivalent or at least not consistently different.

TABLE 2-8: SUMMARY RESULTS OF ACCOMMODATIVE ADAPTATION AS A FUNCTION OF REFRACTIVE GROUP

INVESTIGATOR (YEAR)	DIAGNOSTIC CATEGORIES	N	AGES (yrs.)	APPARATUS	TASK DISTANCE/DURATION	RESULTS
Fisher, Ciuffreda & Levine (1987)	E (±0.75 sph); H (>+0.75sph) low M (>-0.75 and ≤4.00 sph) high M (>-4.00 sph)	48	21-35	Hartinger optometer	accommodative amplitude for 10 min	E=H=low M = high M decay rate: H>E> high & low M
Rosenfield & Gilmartin (1987a)	E (± 0.50 sph & ≤0.50cyl) EOM (-0.50 sph &15y onset) LOM (> -0.50 sph & ≥15y onset)	51	~21	infrared optometer	33 cm, 3.9 & 4.6D for <20sec	E=EOM=LOM
McBrien & Millodot (1988)	E (+0.75 to -0.25sph eq) H (>+0.75 sph eq) EOM (> -0.25 sph eq & ≤13y) LOM (> -0.25 sph eq & ≥15y)	47	18-27	infrared optometer	6, 0.37, 0.20m & TA for 15 min	@.20 & .37cm: LOM> E,EOM>H @6m: LOM> E>EOM>H @ TA: LOM,EOM,E>H
Rosenfield & Gilmartin (1988a)	E (± 0.50 sph & ≤0.50cyl) LOM (>–0.50 & ≤-4.0 sph & ≥15y onset)	20	~22	infrared optometer	33cm with 0, 3 & 6 ΔBO for 3 & 10 min	W/o prisms:E>LOM With prisms: E<LOM Decay rate:E>LOM
Gilmartin, Bullimore, Rosenfield & Winn (1989)	E LOM	30	N.A.	infrared optometer	1,3,5D for 10 min	5D: E>LOM Decay: E>LOM
Gilmartin, Winn, Pugh & Owens (1989)	E LOM	16	N.A.	infrared optometer	3D>TA for 3 min	Decay: E>LOM
Rosenfield & Gilmartin (1989)	E (± 0.50 sph & ≤0.50 cyl) LOM (>-0.50 sph, ≤1cyl & ≥15y onset)	20	~22	infrared optometer	33cm for 15, 30 & 45 sec	E=LOM; Rate of adaptation onset: E=LOM Rate of decay: E=LOM @45s:LOM negative shift

Gilmartin & Bullimore (1991)	E (plano to +0.50 sph eq & ≤0.50 cyl) LOM (-0.50 to -2.25 sph eq & ≤ 0.50 cyl & >15y)	30	19-25	infrared optometer	1, .33 & .20m for 10 min	@1m:LOM>E @.33 & .20m:LOM=E decay rate: @1m: E=LOM @.33 & .20m:LOM>E
Hung & Ciuffreda (1991)	E (± 0.75sph) low M (-0.75 to -4 sph) highM(>-4sph) H (>+0.75sph)	48	21-35	Hartinger coincidence optometer	accommodative amplitude for 10 min	high M>E.H>lowM decay rate: H, low M> high M, E
Harrington, Watanabe, Jiang & White (1992)	E LOM (>15y)	16	N.A.	infrared optometer	6D for 20 min	E=LOM
Miwa & Tokoro (1993a)	<-2 sph > -2 sph	19	19-20	infrared optometer	0.3m with -3D sph for 15 min	hi M> low M
Morse & Smith (1993)	E; LOM EOM	28	N.A.	infrared optometer	4,1,.33 & .20m for 5 min	E=EOM=LOM
Woung, Ukai, Tsuchiya & Ishikawa (1993)	E (+0.75 to -0.25 sph) EOM (>-0.50 sph & ≤ 1cyl & ≤13y) LOM (>- 0.50 sph & ≤ 1cyl & ≥15y)	51	19-38	infrared optometer	4D for 2 min	LOM>E>EOM
Strang, Winn & Gilmartin (1994)	EOM(-0.25 to +0.50 sph & ≤0.50 cyl) LOM(-1.00 to -3.25 sph &≤ 0.50 cyl & >15y onset)	20	23	infrared optometer	3D>TA for 3 min	Rate of decay: E>LOM
Gwiazda, Bauer, Thorn, Held (1995b)	E (+0.75 to -0.25 sph) M (-0.25 to -7.00sph eq) H (+1 to +4.12 sph)	87	6.5-16.5	infrared optometer	4D for 15 min	M>E,H

The slower decay characterizing late-onset myopes was attributed to a reduced sympathetic innervation. This is diametrically opposed to the observation of sympathetically-mediated counteradaptive shifts in late-onset myopes as suggested by the work of Rosenfield and Gilmartin (1989) discussed earlier. Thus, further work in this important area is necessary.

An analogous trend was reported for a group of young children, with myopes showing greater adaptation than either emmetropes or hyperopes (Figure 2-10) (Gwiazda et al. 1995b). Further, myopes of recent onset showed increased adaptation. *Thus, lower tonic accommodation and greater adaptation occurred either during myopia development or its early progression.* These findings are consistent with studies on adults, specifically those between early and late-onset myopes as discussed earlier. Clearly, clinical testing of tonic accommodation and accommodative adaptation need to be advanced and used routinely in the pediatric optometric population, especially for those who are at risk of developing myopia.

Faster post-task adaptation regression for emmetropes relative to late-onset myopes was noted in several studies (Fisher et al. 1987, Rosenfield and Gilmartin 1988a, Gilmartin et al. 1989a, 1989b, Gilmartin and Bullimore 1991, Strang et al. 1994). This difference may be partially accounted for by the relative magnitude of the initial post-task refractive shifts. Fisher et al. (1987) showed that while myopes demonstrated a more prolonged decay relative to the other groups, these differences became statistically insignificant when an analysis of covariance was used to account for the intergroup inequality in the magnitude of the initial accommodative adaptation. Hence, in this case, the longer decay characterizing the myopes was not due to the fact that they have a reduced rate of regression, but rather that they started the decay period at a higher level of accommodative adaptation. Alternatively, the slower regression had also been suggested to reflect a deficit in sympathetic innervation which made them more susceptible to accommodative adaptation (Figure 2-11). Thus, while the regression pattern of emmetropes reflected the normal decay characteristics of the interactive parasympathetic and sympathetic systems, the regression pattern of late-onset myopes appeared to reflect primarily the normal decay of parasympathetic activity alone (Gilmartin and Bullimore 1991).

It has been postulated that the function of the adrenergic innervation was the attenuation of the magnitude and duration of the accommodative adaptation (Gilmartin and Hogan 1985b, Gilmartin and Bullimore 1987). Studies using timolol which effectively blocked beta-2 receptors enhanced the adaptation as well as extended the decay time course five to tenfold (Gilmartin and Bullimore 1987). This sympathetically-mediated mechanism was proposed to be responsible for the absence of shifts in emmetropes and early-onset myopes, as well as for inducing counteradaptive shifts in

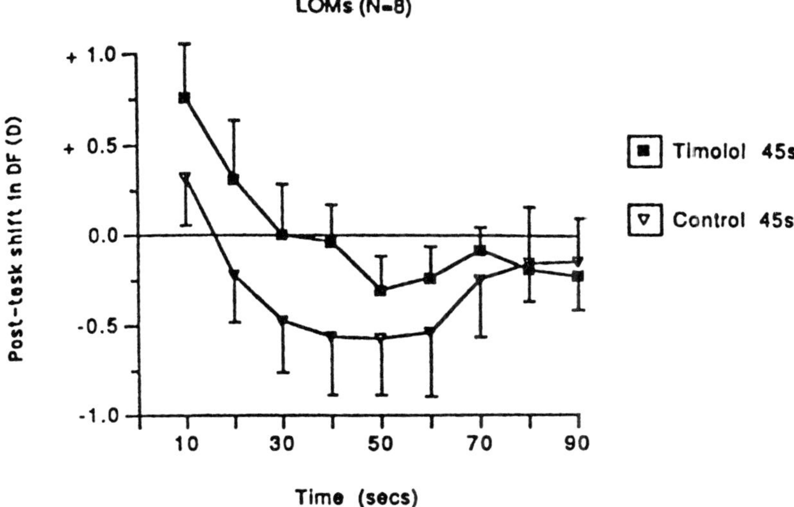

Figure 2-9 : Effect of timolol maleate (0.5%) on the mean post-task dioptric shift in dark focus against time for 8 late-onset myopes after a 45s near-vision task. The control data indicate the regression of dark focus for the same subjects in the absence of timolol. Error bars represent ± 1 SEM (Reprinted with permission, Rosenfield and Gilmartin 1989).

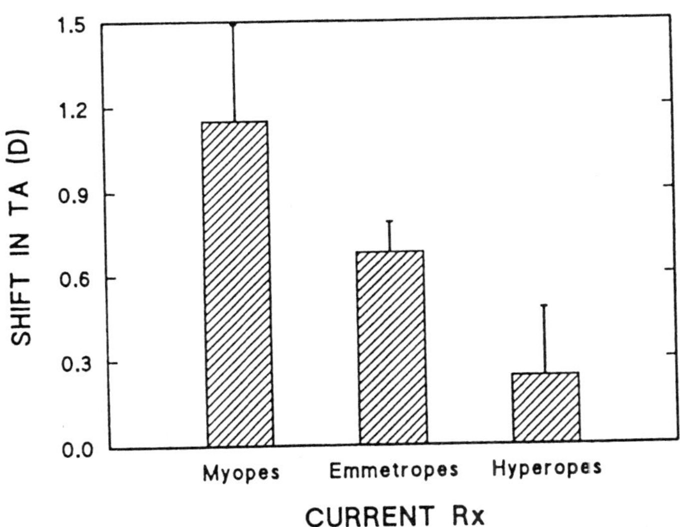

Figure 2-10 : Mean dioptric shift in tonic accommodation after 15 min of near focus for myopic, emmetropic and hyperopic children; bars show standard errors (Reprinted with permission, Gwiazda et al. 1995b).

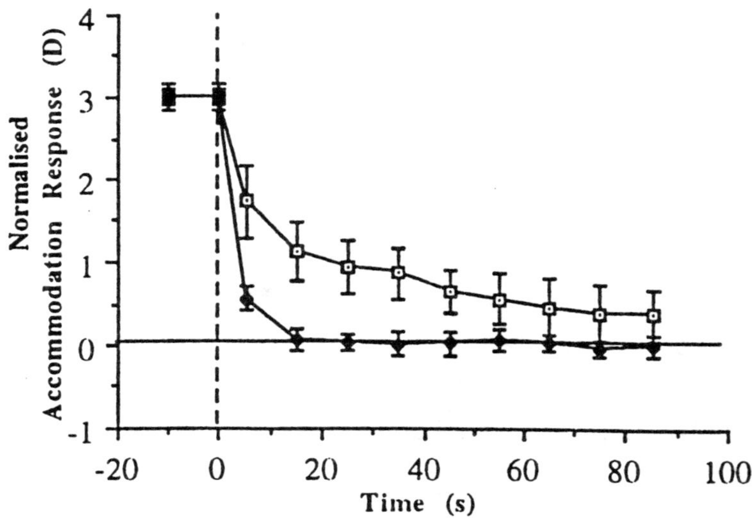

Figure 2-11 : Differences in regression patterns are shown for group data in emmetropes (•) and late onset myopes (□). The mean data for each groups were averaged. Error bars represent 2 SEMs. Subjects fixated an illuminated 3D target which was subsequently extinguished, and the decay to the pre-task tonic accommodative level was monitored objectively. (Reprinted with permission, Strang et al. 1994).

hyperopes at near (McBrien and Millodot 1988). Its deficit adversely affected adaptation. Furthermore, the relative strength of the dual autonomic innervation possibly accounted for the difference between groups, and furthermore, that this variation in adaptation was primarily due to variations in the sympathetic component (McBrien and Millodot 1988). Thus, reduced sympathetic input yielded increased adaptive shifts at near and an absence of hyperopic shifts at far. This explanation also appears to be consistent with data on the regression of adaptation. The authors further made the inference that hyperopes had greater parasympathetic, while late-onset myopes had less parasympathetic innervation. Indeed, reduced tonic accommodation in myopes had been documented and discussed in the previous section. Further, an inverse relation between tonic accommodation and its adaptation has been postulated (Morse and Smith 1993, Ebenholtz 1985, Gilmartin and Bullimore 1987, Owens and Wolf-Kelly 1987). It was suggested that a low tonic accommodation resulted in increased adaptation, and hence myopes who were characterized with possessing low tonic accommodative levels were predisposed to a greater amount of adaptation. Gilmartin and Bullimore (1987) also showed that the characteristics of accommodative adaptation varied with the level of pre-task tonic accommodation. For pre-task tonic accommodation >0.55D (Figure 2-12a), decay was complete within

(a)

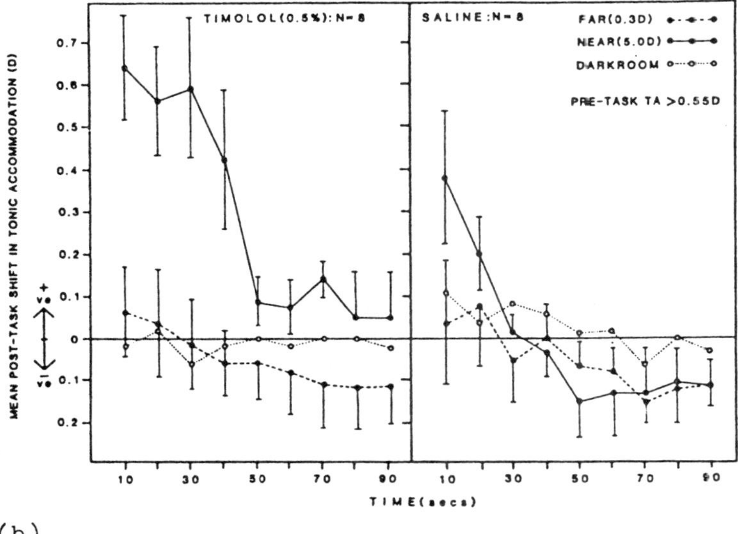

(b)

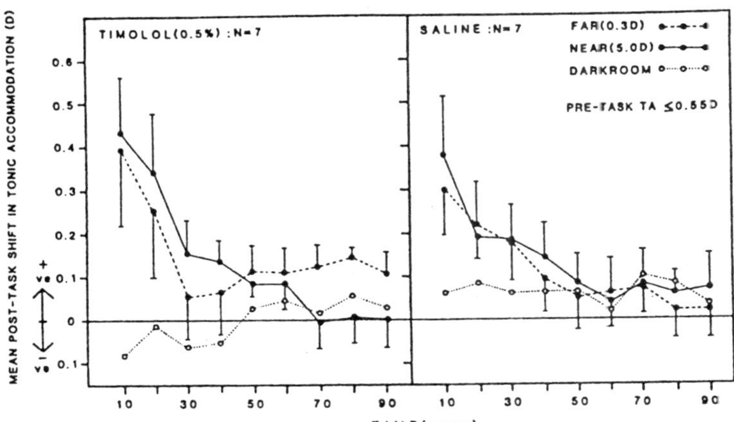

Figure 2-12 : (a) Mean post-task dioptric shift in tonic accommodation (TA) against time for each experimental condition and for the group of 8 subjects having pre-task TA levels >0.55D (N.B. the pre-task TA value does not include the +0.20D calibration factor). Error bars represent ± 1 SEM.
(b) Mean post-task dioptric shift in tonic accommodation (TA) against time for each experimental condition and for the group of 7 subjects having pre-task TA levels ≤ 0.55D (N.B. the pre-task TA value does not include the +0.20D calibration factor). Error bars represent ± 1 SEM (Reprinted with permission, Gilmartin and Bullimore 1987).

30-40s due to the presence of both autonomic components. Moreover, a counteradaptive shift was evident after 20s. This was once again attributed to sympathetically-mediated inhibition which can be eliminated by timolol. In fact, following the instillation of timolol, increased adaptation was apparent. On the other hand, for pre-task tonic accommodation <0.55D (Figure 2-12b), no negative shifts were demonstrated. Timolol failed to induce any effect, further supporting the notion of a lack of sympathetic innervation in these individuals. Thus, these same individuals were more susceptible to adaptation.

The association between accommodative adaptation and myopic development has been debated over the years. Excessive and cumulative adaptation had been suggested to act as precursors to myopia (Gilmartin and Bullimore 1991). For example, if the accommodative adaptation magnitude did not decay rapidly to pre-task baseline following disengagement of one's near focusing activity, with successive periods of near work, this residual accommodation could "accumulate" resulting in a closer far point, i.e., pseudo or perhaps even permanent myopia. Persistent and maintained adaptation resulting from a sympathetic deficit could also be a predisposing factor (Gilmartin et al. 1989b).

Nearwork-Induced Transient Myopia

Nearwork-induced transient myopia (NITM) refers to the transient pseudomyopic shift in the far point of the eye occurring in the presence of blur following relatively brief periods of nearwork (Ong and Ciuffreda 1995). A limited number of studies have investigated NITM as a function of refractive group (Fisher et al. 1987, Harrington et al. 1992, Miwa and Tokoro 1993a). In one study (Miwa and Tokoro 1993a), similar amounts of NITM were found in the various refractive groups, whereas in the other two investigations (Fisher et al. 1987, Harrington et al. 1992), no NITM was found (Table 2-9). This may in part be related to the relatively small sample sizes used which inevitably reduced statistical power. For example, although Fisher et al. (1987) reported NITM for the whole sample group, no such NITM was demonstrated for each refractive subgroup. Furthermore, the finding of a lack of relation between NITM and refraction may also be attributed to the methodology. For example, Harrington et al. (1992) did not find any evidence of differential NITM. However, it appeared that their post-task measurement of refraction was not obtained immediately following completion of the near task. Thus, it is likely that any adaptation effects which might have occurred had already decayed to baseline, as it is unusual not to find any adaptation whatsoever. However, ongoing investigations in our laboratory clearly demonstrate that myopes are much more susceptible to NITM than either emmetropes or hyperopes. Also see Chapter 4.

DYNAMIC ACCOMMODATION

Accommodation typically responds to a change in blur stimulus following a latency of 360 ms from far-to-near and 380 ms from near-to-far (Campbell and Westheimer 1960). Actual lens movement time is 640 ms from far-to-near and 560 ms from near-to-far (Campbell and Westheimer 1960). Therefore, it takes approximately one second from stimulus onset to attain the final accommodative single response amplitude. The average peak velocity reported for a 2D step stimulus is 10D/s, with this velocity increasing as a function of stimulus magnitude (Schnider et al. 1984, Ciuffreda and Kruger 1988, Hung and Ciuffreda 1988, Mordi 1991).

There are few studies of accommodative dynamics as a function of refractive group. Suzumura (1979) objectively recorded dynamic accommodative responses in 126 eyes (Table 2-10). More specifically, the latency, speed, and frequency spectrum of accommodative oscillations were studied as a target was alternated between far and near positions. A refraction-dependent trend seemed evident for latency, with it being longer for hyperopes (431ms) than for either myopes (393 ms) or emmetropes (327 ms). However, the values were all within normal limits (Campbell and Westheimer 1960, Ciuffreda 1991, in press). There was also an apparent difference for average accommodative velocity, with it being faster for emmetropes (5.69 D/t) than either myopes (2.84 D/t) or hyperopes (1.47D/t). In other words, the average velocity of the myopes was approximately half that of the emmetropes and twice that of the hyperopes. However, since the accommodative response amplitudes for the emmetropes and myopes were noticeably larger than for the hyperopes, their maximum velocity would be predicted to be higher due to the "main sequence" neurological control of accommodation in which accommodative peak velocity is proportional to accommodative response amplitude (Ciuffreda and Kruger 1988). In addition, investigation of accommodative microfluctuations showed that the high frequency component (>2Hz) was more evident in emmetropes and myopes than in hyperopes. However, recent evidence (Winn et al. 1990) suggests the high frequency oscillations are primarily biological noise related to the arterial pulse and not to direct (or indirect) visual feedback related to accommodation. Similarly, Zhai and Guan (1988) assessed accommodation dynamics in a sample of 128 students aged 10 to 19 years. They reported that accommodative reaction time was also significantly increased in myopes relative to emmetropes. This was true for both increasing (2.11 versus 1.82s) and decreasing (1.64 versus 1.13s) total accommodative response time. In addition, the speed of the accommodative response was also slower in myopes (5.64 versus 8.76 D/s for decreasing accommodation and 4.37 versus 5.24 D/s for increasing accommodation).

TABLE 2-9: SUMMARY RESULTS OF NEARWORK-INDUCED TRANSIENT MYOPIA AS A FUNCTION OF REFRACTIVE GROUP

INVESTIGATOR (YEAR)	DIAGNOSTIC CATEGORIES	N	AGES (yrs.)	APPARATUS	TASK/CONDITIO N	RESULTS
Fisher, Ciuffreda & Levine (1987)	E (±0.75 sph) H (>+0.75 sph) low M (>-0.75 & ≤-4.00 sph) high M (>-4.00 sph)	48	21-35	Hartinger optometer	monocular @ accommodative amplitude for 10 min	E=H=low M =high M
Harrington, Watanabe, Jiang & White (1992)	E LOM (>15y)	16	N.A.	infrared optometer	play computer game @ 6D for 20 min	E=LOM
Miwa & Tokoro (1993a)	<-2 sph >-2 sph	19	19-20	infrared optometer	binocularly read magazine @ 0.3m w/-3 sph for 15 min	low M = high M

TABLE 2-10: SUMMARY RESULTS OF DYNAMIC ACCOMMODATION AS A FUNCTION OF REFRACTIVE GROUP

INVESTIGATOR (YEAR)	DIAGNOSTIC CATEGORIES	N	AGES (yrs.)	APPARATUS	RESULTS
Suzumura (1979)	E, H & M	126 eyes	5-49	dynamic infrared optometer	latency: H>M>E; speed: E>M>H
Zhai & Guan (1988)	E (+0.50 to -0.25 sph) M (-1 to -3 sph & 0.5 cyl)	256 eyes	10-19	dynamic accommodo-polyrecorder	reaction time: M>E; speed: E>M
Storey, Tromans & Rabie (1990)	E (+1 to -0.50 sph) M (-2.50 to -9 sph & <1 cyl)	24	18-30	dynamic biometry	response time: (@ 2 & 4D): E>M (@ 6D): M>E
Schaeffel, Wilhelm & Zrenner (1993)	E, LOM	19	25-33	dynamic infrared optometer	speed: E=LOM

In contrast, Storey et al. (1990) performed continuous ultrasonic biometry on 24 emmetropes and myopes. The accommodative stimulus was varied between 2, 4, and 6D. The mean response time for changes in the anterior chamber and lens was greater for emmetropes at stimulus levels of 2 and 4D and for myopes at the 6D stimulus level. On the other hand, Schaeffel et al. (1993) objectively recorded accommodation in 19 subjects. There was no relation between accommodative peak velocity and refractive state. However, the sample size was relatively small, and the refractive distribution extremely unequal. Only a handful of subjects (5/19) had refractive errors greater than ± 1D. Of these, three were myopes and two were hyperopes. Testing on such a kurtotic subject sample would presumably result in reduced differences between groups, that is, if any existed at all. Clearly, further work is needed in this area.

SUMMARY

From the foregoing, it is evident that the multitude of investigations on the different aspects of accommodation as they relate to refractive error have proven to be inconclusive in many cases. According to Goss and Zhai (1995), some of the discrepancies can be partially accounted for by the lack of uniformity in subjects' ages, the unequal refractive error distribution, the difference in refractive criterion, instrumentation, and the use of different reference planes in the assessment of accommodation. In view of some of the inconsistency in data, the following is an attempt to consolidate and summarize the general trends (based on our opinion in determining the more credible and problem-free data presented) towards the end of drawing some degree of closure to this confusing area. See Tables 2-1 to 2-10 for specifics of the experiments and Table 2-11 for a qualitative summary of refractive group accommodative response relative to emmetropes.

(1) *Accommodative stimulus/response function:* The majority of the studies found reduced steady-state accommodative responsivity at near in myopes.

(2) *Accommodative amplitude:* Results on accommodative amplitude have been equivocal. Almost half of the studies indicated an absence of differences between refractive groups, while the other half reported greater accommodative amplitude for either myopes or emmetropes.

(3) *Convergent accommodation:* Convergent accommodation was consistently found to be similar between emmetropes and myopes.

(4) *Disparity-induced accommodation:* Disparity-induced accommodation was found to be increased in late-onset myopes versus emmetropes.

(5) *AC/A ratio*: Most studies showed increased AC/A for myopes relative to hyperopes and emmetropes.

(6) *Proximally-induced accommodation*: Emmetropes exhibited increased proximally-induced accommodation relative to late-onset myopes.

(7) *Tonic accommodation*: Although the results are equivocal, nonetheless, the majority of them indicated that myopes exhibited reduced tonic accommodation relative to the other refractive groups.

(8) *Accommodative adaptation*: The results on accommodative adaptation are somewhat equivocal. Its initial magnitude had been demonstrated to be either similar across refractive groups or perhaps show an increase in myopes. On the other hand, refractive group-related differential decay rates were reported by the vast majority of the studies, with the slowest decay being evident for myopes.

(9) *Nearwork-induced transient myopia*: With the exception of our ongoing investigation, all other studies in this area consistently found no difference in transient myopia between refractive groups, although most studies did not even report the occurrence ofNITM which is highly unusual..

(10*) Dynamic accommodation:* Accommodative latency was found to be greatest in hyperopes followed by myopes and emmetropes. Its speed was noted to be greatest for emmetropes followed by myopes and hyperopes in most studies.

TABLE 2-11: SUMMARY OF ACCOMMODATIVE CHARACTERISTICS AS A FUNCTION OF REFRACTIVE GROUP RELATIVE TO EMMETROPES*

ACCOMMODATIVE PARAMETER	LOM	EOM	H
Static Aspects			
Accommodative stimulus/response	↓	↓	↓,↑,=
Accommodative amplitude	↑	↑,=	=
Convergent accommodation	=	=	
Disparity-induced accommodation	↑	=	
AC/A ratio	↑	↑	
Proximally-induced accommodation	↓		
Tonic accommodation	↓	=	↑,=
Accommodative adaptation	↑	=	↓
Rate of onset	=		
Rate of decay	↓		
Nearwork-induced transient myopia	↑	↑	=
Dynamic Aspects			
Latency			↑
Speed	=		↓

Table legend:
LOM = late-onset myopes
EOM = early-onset myopes
H = hyperopes
↑ = increased relative to emmetropes
↓ = decreased relative to emmetropes
= represents similar responses to emmetropes.

*Data on myopes in general, with no distinction between early and late onset, were not included.

REFERENCES

Adams DW, McBrien NA. A longitudinal study of the relationship between tonic accommodation (dark focus) and refractive error in adulthood. Invest Ophthalmol Vis Sci (Suppl). 1993; 34: 1308.

Alpern M. Vergence and accommodation. I. Can change in size induce vergence movements? Arch Ophthalmol. 1958; 60: 355-7.

Alpern M, Kincaid WM, Lubeck MJ. Vergence and accommodation. III. Proposed definitions of the ACA ratios. Am J Ophthalmol. 1959; 48: 141-8.

Alpern M, Larson BF. Vergence and accommodation. IV. Effect of luminance quantity on the AC/A. Am J Ophthalmol. 1960; 49: 1140-9.

Baldwin WR. Accommodative characteristics of a group of myopic adults. Am J Optom Arch Am Acad Optom. 1965; 42: 237-43.

Birnbaum MH. Nearpoint visual stress: Clinical implications. J Am Optom Assoc. 1985; 56: 480-90.

Blustein GH, Rosenfield M, Ciuffreda KJ. Does dark accommodation really change following sustained near fixation? Optom Vis Sci (Suppl). 1993; 70: 16.

Borish IM. Clinical refraction, 3rd ed. Chicago: Professional Press, Inc.; 1970.

Braddick O, Ayling L, Sawyer R, Atkinson J. A photorefractive study of dark focus and refraction. Vis Res. 1981; 21: 1761-4.

Breinin GW, Chin NB. Accommodation, convergence and aging. Doc Ophthalmol. 1972; 34: 109-21.

Bullimore MA, Boyd T, Mather HE, Gilmartin B. Near retinoscopy and refractive error. Clin Exp Optom. 1988; 71: 114-8.

Bullimore MA, Gilmartin B. Aspects of tonic accommodation in emmetropia and late-onset myopia. Am J Optom Physiol Opt. 1987; 64: 499-503.

Bullimore MA, Gilmartin B. The accommodative response, refractive error and mental effort: 1. The sympathetic nervous system. Doc Ophthalmol. 1988; 69: 385-97.

Bullimore MA, Gilmartin B, Royston JM. Steady-state accommodation and ocular biometry in late-onset myopia. Doc Ophthalmol. 1992; 80: 143-55.

Campbell FW, Westheimer G. Dynamics of accommodation responses of the human eye. J Physiol. 1960; 151: 285-95.

Carreras MM. La miopia nocturna e influencia sobre la misma de la amplitud de acomodacion. Arch Soc Oftal Hisp Am. 1951; 11: 1443-89. Cited in Charman WN. The accommodative resting point and refractive error. Ophthal Optician. 1982; 21: 469-73.

Charman WN. The accommodative resting point and refractive error. Ophthal Optician. 1982; 21: 469-73.

Ciuffreda KJ. Accommodation and its anomalies. In: Charman WN, ed. Visual optics and instrumentation: vision and visual dysfunction, Vol. 1. London: MacMillan; 1991: 231-79.

Ciuffreda KJ. Components of clinical near vergence testing. J Behavioral Optom. 1992; 3: 3-13.

Ciuffreda KJ. Accommodation, pupil, and presbyopia. In: Borish IM, Benjamin J, eds. Clinical refraction:principles and practice. Philadelphia: Saunders; in press.

Ciuffreda KJ, Kenyon RV. Accommodative vergence and accommodation in normals, amblyopes, and strabismics. In: Schor CM, Ciuffreda KJ, eds. Vergence eye movements: basic and clinical aspects. Boston: Butterworth; 1983: 101-73.

Ciuffreda KJ, Kruger PB. Dynamics of human voluntary accommodation. Am J Optom Physiol Opt. 1988; 65: 365-70.

Duane A. Normal values of the accommodation at all ages. J Am Med Assn. 1912; 59: 1010-3.

Ebenholtz SM. Accommodative hysteresis: a precursor for induced myopia? Invest Ophthalmol Vis Sci. 1983; 24: 513-5.
Ebenholtz SM. Accommodative hysteresis: relation to resting focus. Am J Optom Physiol Opt. 1985; 62: 755-62.
Fisher SK, Ciuffreda KJ, Bird JE. The effect of stimulus duration on tonic accommodation and tonic vergence. Optom Vis Sci. 1990; 67: 441-9.
Fisher SK, Ciuffreda KJ, Levine S. Tonic accommodation, accommodative hysteresis and refractive error. Am J Optom Physiol Opt. 1987; 64: 799-809.
Fledelius HC. Accommodation and juvenile myopia. Doc Ophthal Proc Series. 1981; 28: 103-8.
Flom MC, Takahashi E. The AC/A ratio and undercorrected myopia. Am J Optom Arch Am Acad Optom. 1962; 39: 305-12.
Francois J, Goes F. Comparative study of ultrasonic biometry of emmetropes and myopes with special regard to the heredity of myopia. In: Gitter KA, Keeney AH, Sarin LK, Meyer D, eds. Ophthalmic ultrasound-proceedings of the 4th international congress of ultrasonography in ophthalmology, Philadelphia. St. Louis: C.V. Mosby Co., 1969: 165-80.
Garner LF. Mechanisms of accommodation and refractive error. Ophthal Physiol Opt. 1983; 3: 287-93.
Garner LF, Yap M, Scott R. Crystalline lens power in myopia. Optom Vis Sci. 1992; 69: 863-865.
Gawron VJ. Differences among myopes, emmetropes, and hyperopes. Am J Optom Physiol Opt. 1981; 58: 753-60.
Gilmartin B, Bullimore MA. Sustained near-vision augments inhibitory sympathetic innervation of the ciliary muscle. Clin Vis Sci. 1987; 1: 197-208.
Gilmartin B, Bullimore MA. Adaptation of tonic accommodation to sustained visual tasks in emmetropia and late-onset myopia. Optom Vis Sci. 1991; 68: 22-6.
Gilmartin B, Bullimore MA, Rosenfield M, Winn B. Ciliary muscle tonus and innervation in late-onset myopia. Invest Ophthalmol Vis Sci (Suppl). 1989a; 30: 325.
Gilmartin B, Hogan RE. The relationship between tonic accommodation and ciliary muscle innervation. Invest Ophthalmol Vis Sci. 1985a; 26: 1024-8.
Gilmartin B, Hogan RE. The role of sympathetic nervous system in ocular accommodation and ametropia. Ophthal Physiol Opt. 1985b; 5: 91-3.
Gilmartin B, Winn B, Pugh JR, Owens H. Ciliary muscle innervation and predisposition to late-onset myopia. Optom Vis Sci (Suppl). 1989b; 66: 217.
Goss DA, Zhai H. Clinical and laboratory investigations of the relationship of accommodation and convergence function with refractive error - a literature review. Doc Ophthalmol. 1994; 86: 349-80.
Grant V. Accommodation and convergence in visual space perception. J Exp Psychol. 1942; 31: 89-104.
Gwiazda J, Bauer J, Thorn F, Held R. A dynamic relationship between myopia and blur-driven accommodation in school-aged children. Vis Res. 1995a; 35: 1299-304.
Gwiazda J, Bauer J, Thorn F, Held R. Shifts in tonic accommodation after near work are related to refractive errors in children. Ophthal Physiol Opt. 1995b; 15: 93-7.
Gwiazda J, Thorn F, Bauer J, Held R. Myopic children show insufficient accommodative response to blur. Invest Ophthalmol Vis Sci. 1993; 34: 690-4.
Hamasaki D, Ong J, Marg E. The amplitude of accommodation in presbyopia. Am J Optom Arch Am Acad Optom. 1956; 33: 3-14.
Harrington S, Watanabe DS, Jiang BC, White JM. Accommodative adaptation does not alter the accommodative stimulus/response function. Optom Vis Sci (Suppl). 1992; 69: 110.

Held R, Gwiazda JE, Thorn F, Bauer JA. Changes in accommodative responsiveness are linked to the development of myopia in children. Invest Ophthalmol Vis Sci (Suppl). 1994; 35: 1735.

Hennessy RT, Leibowitz HW. The effect of peripheral stimulus on accommodation. Percept Psychophys. 1971; 10: 129-32.

Heron G, Bahri PK, Burnside JA, Kacouli K, Mackintosh SR. The relation between dark focus of accommodation and refractive error. Ophthal Physiol Opt. 1984; 4: 187.

Hofstetter HW. A comparison of Duane's and Donders' tables of the amplitude of accommodation. Am J Optom Arch Am Acad Optom. 1944; 21: 345-63.

Hung GK, Ciuffreda KJ. Dual-mode behaviour in the human accommodation system. Ophthal Physiol Opt. 1988; 8: 327-32.

Hung GK, Ciuffreda KJ. Model of tonic accommodation after sustained near focus. Optom Vis Sci. 1991; 68: 617-23.

Hung GK, Ciuffreda KJ, Rosenfield M. Proximal contribution to a linear static model of accommodation and vergence. Ophthal Physiol Opt. 1996; 16: 31-41.

Hung GK, Semmlow JL. Static behavior of accommodation and vergence: computer simulation of an interactive dual-feedback system. IEEE Trans Biomed Engn. 1980; BME-27: 439-47.

Irving A. Ametropia at low illuminations, MSc Thesis, University of Manchester (Technology), 1957. Cited in Charman WN. The accommodative resting point and refractive error. Ophthal Optician. 1982; 21: 469-73.

Ittleson WH, Ames A. Accommodation, convergence and their relation to apparent distance. J Psychol. 1950; 30: 43-62.

Jaschinski-Kruza W, Toenies U. Effect of a mental arithmetic task on dark focus of accommodation. Ophthal Physiol Opt. 1988; 8: 432-7.

Jiang BC. Parameters of accommodative and vergence systems and the development of late-onset myopia. Invest Ophthalmol Vis Sci. 1995; 36: 1737-42.

Johnson CA, Post RB, Chalupa LM, Lee TJ. Monocular deprivation in humans: a study of identical twins. Invest Ophthalmol Vis Sci. 1982; 23: 135-8.

Jones R. Accommodative and convergence control system parameters are abnormal in myopia. Invest Ophthalmol Vis Sci (Suppl). 1990; 31: 81.

Jones R. The effect of proximal accommodation on accommodative accuracy. Optom Vis Sci (Suppl). 1993; 70: 56.

Kelly TS-B. Myopia or expansion glaucoma. In: Fledelius HC, Alsbirk PH, Goldschmidt E, eds. Third International Conference on Myopia. The Hague: Dr W. Junk Publishers. Doc Ophthal Proc Series. 1981; 28: 109-16.

Kotulak JC, Schor CM. The effects of optical vergence, contrast, and luminance on the accommodative response to spatially bandpass filtered targets. Vis Res. 1987; 27: 1797-806.

Kruger PB, Pola J. Changing target size is a stimulus for accommodation. J Opt Soc Am. 1985; 2: 1832-5.

Leibowitz HW, Owens DA. New evidence for the intermediate position of relaxed accommodation. Doc Ophthalmol. 1978; 46: 133-47.

Maddock RJ, Millodot M, Leat S, Johnson C. Accommodation responses and refractive error. Invest Ophthalmol Vis Sci. 1981; 20: 387-91.

Manas L. The inconstancy of the ACA ratio. Am J Optom Arch Am Acad Optom. 1955; 32: 304-15.

McBrien NA, Millodot M. Amplitude of accommodation and refractive error. Invest Ophthalmol Vis Sci. 1986a; 27: 1187-90.

McBrien NA, Millodot M.The effect of refractive error on the accommodative response gradient. Ophthal Physiol Opt. 1986b; 6:145-9.

McBrien NA, Millodot M. The relationship between tonic accommodation and refractive error. Invest Ophthalmol Vis Sci. 1987; 28:997-1004.

McBrien NA, Millodot M. Differences in adaptation of tonic accommodation with refractive state. Invest Ophthalmol Vis Sci. 1988; 29: 460-9.

Miwa T. Instrument myopia and the resting state of accommodation. Optom Vis Sci. 1992; 69: 55-9.

Miwa T, Tokoro T. Accommodative hysteresis of refractive errors in light and dark fields. Optom Vis Sci. 1993a; 70: 323-7.

Miwa T, Tokoro T. Relation between the dark focus of accommodation and refractive error-a cycloplegic study. Optom Vis Sci. 1993b; 70: 328-31.

Mordi JA. Accommodation, aging and presbyopia. PhD thesis, SUNY/State College of Optometry, New York; 1991.

Morgan MW, Jr. Accommodation and its relationship to convergence. Am J Optom Arch Am Acad Optom. 1944; 21: 183-95.

Morgan MW. Effect of perceived distance on accommodation and convergence. In Trans internat ophthalmic optical congress. New York : Hafner Pub. Co.; 1962: 3-15.

Morgan MW. Accommodation and vergence. Am J Optom Arch Am Acad Optom. 1968a; 45: 415-54.

Morgan MW. Stimulus to and response of accommodation. Can J Optom. 1968b; 30: 71-8.

Morse SE, Smith EL III. Long-term adaptational aftereffects of accommodation are associated with distal dark focus and not with late onset myopia. Invest Ophthalmol Vis Sci (Suppl). 1993; 34: 1308.

Newman FA. Acquired axial myopia. Am J Ophthalmol. 1929; 12: 714-9.

Ni J, Smith EL III. Effects of chronic optical defocus on the kitten's refractive status. Vis Res. 1989; 29: 929-38.

Ong E, Ciuffreda KJ, Tannen B. Static accommodation in congenital nystagmus. Invest Ophthalmol Vis Sci. 1993; 34: 194-204.

Owens DA, Harris D, Owens RL, Francis EL. Tonic accommodation and late-onset myopia: a longitudinal investigation. Invest Ophthalmol Vis Sci (Suppl). 1989; 30: 325.

Owens RL, Higgins KE. Long term stability of the dark focus of accommodation. Am J Optom Physiol Opt. 1983; 60: 32-8.

Owens DA, Wolf-Kelly K. Near work, visual fatigue, and variations of oculomotor tonus. Invest Ophthalmol Vis Sci. 1987; 28: 743-9.

Post RB, Johnson CA, Owens DA. Does performance of tasks affect the resting focus of accommodation? Am J Optom Physiol Opt. 1985; 62: 533-7.

Post RB, Johnson CA, Tsuetaki TK. Comparison of laser and infrared techniques for measurement of the resting focus of accommodation: mean differences and long-term variability. Ophthal Physiol Opt .1984; 4: 327-32.

Rabin J, Van Sluyters RC, Malach R. Emmetropization: a vision-dependent phenomenon. Invest Ophthalmol Vis Sci. 1981; 20: 561-4.

Ramsdale C. Monocular and binocular accommodation. Ophthal Optician. 1979; 19: 606-22.

Ramsdale C. The effect of ametropia on the accommodative response. Acta Ophthalmol. 1985; 63: 167-74.

Ripple PH. Variation of accommodation in vertical directions of gaze. Am J Ophthalmol. 1952; 35: 1630-4.

Rosenfield M. Comparison of accommodative adaptation using laser and infra-red optometers. Ophthal Physiol Opt. 1989; 9: 431-6.

Rosenfield M, Ciuffreda KJ. Proximal and cognitively-induced accommodation. Ophthal Physiol Opt. 1990; 10: 252-6.

Rosenfield M, Ciuffreda KJ. Effect of surround propinquity on the open-loop accommodative response. Invest Ophthalmol Vis Sci 1991; 32: 142-147.
Rosenfield M, Ciuffreda KJ, Hung GK. The linearity of proximally-induced accommodation and vergence. Invest Ophthalmol Vis Sci. 1991; 32: 2985-91.
Rosenfield M, Ciuffreda KJ, Hung GK, Gilmartin B. Tonic accommodation: a review. I. Basic aspects. Ophthal Physiol Opt. 1993; 13: 266-84.
Rosenfield M, Ciuffreda KJ, Hung GK, Gilmartin B. Tonic accommodation: a review. II. Accommodative adaptation and clinical aspects. Ophthal Physiol Opt. 1994; 14: 1-13.
Rosenfield M, Ciuffreda KJ, Ong E, Azimi A. Proximally induced accommodation and adaptation. Invest Ophthalmol Vis Sci. 1990; 31: 1162-1167.
Rosenfield M, Gilmartin B. Effect of a near-vision task on the response AC/A of a myopic population. Ophthal Physiol Opt. 1987a; 7: 225-33.
Rosenfield M, Gilmartin B. Synkinesis of accommodation and vergence in late-onset myopia. Am J Optom Physiol Opt. 1987c; 64: 929-37.
Rosenfield M, Gilmartin B. Accommodative adaptation induced by sustained disparity-vergence. Am J Optom Physiol Opt. 1988a; 65: 118-26.
Rosenfield M, Gilmartin B. Assessment of the CA/C ratio in a myopic population. Am J Optom Physiol Opt. 1988b; 65: 168-73.
Rosenfield M, Gilmartin B. Disparity-induced accommodation in late-onset myopia. Ophthal Physiol Opt. 1988c; 8: 353-5.
Rosenfield M, Gilmartin B. Temporal aspects of accommodative adaptation. Optom Vis Sci. 1989; 66: 229-34.
Rosenfield M, Gilmartin B. Effect of target proximity on the open-loop accommodative response. Optom Vis Sci. 1990; 67: 74-9.
Rosner J, Rosner J. Relation between clinically measured tonic accommodation and refractive status in 6- to 14-year-old children. Optom Vis Sci. 1989; 66: 436-9.
Sato T. The causes and prevention of acquired myopia. Yokohama: Helarudo Printing Co., Ltd.; 1957.
Schaeffel F, Wilhelm H, Zrenner E. Inter-individual variability in the dynamics of natural accommodation in humans: Relation to age and refractive errors. J Physiol. 1993; 461: 301-20.
Schnider CM, Ciuffreda KJ, Cooper J, Kruger PB. Accommodation dynamics in divergence excess exotropia. Invest Ophthalmol Vis Sci. 1984; 25: 414-8.
Schor CM, Kotulak JC. Dynamic interactions between accommodation and convergence are velocity sensitive. Vis Res. 1986; 26: 927-42.
Schor CM, Kotulak JC, Tsuetaki T. Adaptation of tonic accommodation reduces accommodative lag and is masked in darkness. Invest Ophthalmol Vis Sci. 1986; 27: 820-7.
Simonelli NM. The dark focus of the human eye and its relationship to age and visual defect. Hum Factors. 1983; 25: 85-92.
Smith G. The accommodative resting states, instrument accommodation and their measurement. Optica Acta. 1983; 30: 347-59.
Stenström S. Investigation of the variation and the correlation of the optical elements of human eyes, trans. by Woolf D. Am J Optom Arch Am Acad Optom. 1948; 25: 218-32, 286-99, 340-50, 388-97, 438-49, 496-504.
Storey JK, Rabie EP. Ultrasound- a research tool in the study of accommodation. Ophthal Physiol Opt. 1983; 3: 315-20.
Storey JK, Tromans C, Rabie E. Continuous biometry of the crystalline lens during accommodation. In: Sampaolesi R, ed. Ultrasonography in ophthalmology. Dordrecht: Kluwer Academic Publishers; 1990: 117-23.
Strang NC, Winn B, Gilmartin B. Repeatability of post-task regression of accommodation in emmetropia and late-onset myopia. Ophthal Physiol Opt. 1994; 14: 88-91.

Suzumura A. Accommodation in myopia. J Aiche Med Univ Ass. 1979; 7: 6-15.
Toates FM. A model of accommodation. Vis Res. 1970; 10: 1069-76.
Toates FM. Accommodative function of the human eye. Physiol Rev. 1972; 52: 828-63.
Tokoro T. The role of accommodation in myopia. Acta Ophthalmologica (Suppl). 1988; 185: 153-5.
Tornqvist G. The relative importance of the parasympathetic and sympathetic nervous systems for accommodation in monkeys. Invest Ophthalmol Vis Sci. 1967; 6: 612-7.
Tsuetaki TK, Schor CM. Clinical method for measuring adaptation of tonic accommodation and vergence accommodation. Am J Optom Physiol Opt. 1987; 64: 437-49.
Turner MJ. Observations on the normal subjective amplitude of accommodation. Br J Physiol Opt. 1958; 15: 70-100.
Van Alphen GWHM. On emmetropia and ametropia. Ophthalmologica (Suppl). 1961; 142: 1-92.
Wallman J, Gottlieb MD, Rajaram V, Fugate-Wentzek LA. Local retinal regions control local eye growth and myopia. Science. 1987; 237: 73-7.
Wesson MD, Koenig R. A new clinical method for direct measurement of fixation disparity. South J Optom. 1983; 1: 48-52.
Wiesel TN, Raviola E. Myopia and eye enlargement after neonatal lid fusion in monkeys. Nature. 1977; 266: 66-7.
Winn B, Gilmartin B, Mortimer LC, Edwards NR. The effect of mental effort on open- and closed-loop accommodation. Ophthal Physiol Opt. 1991; 11: 335-9.
Winn B, Pugh JR, Gilmartin B, Owens H. Arterial pulse modulates steady-state ocular accommodation. Curr Eye Res. 1990; 9: 971-5.
Wolf KS, Ciuffreda KJ, Jacobs SE. Time course and decay of effects of near work on tonic accommodation and tonic vergence. Optom Vis Sci. 1987; 7: 131-5.
Woung LC, Ukai K, Tsuchiya K, Ishikawa S. Accommodative adaptation and age of onset of myopia. Ophthal Physiol Opt. 1993; 13: 366-70.
Zhai H, Guan Z. Observation of accommodation in juvenile myopia. Eye Sci. 1988; 4: 228-31.

FOOTNOTE

Congruent conditions represent equidioptric accommodative and vergence stimulus conditions, while non-congruent conditions represent unequal accommodative and vergence stimulus demands. When one looks at a target at 40cm with full optical correction, the accommodative and vergence stimuli are equal and numerically equivalent to 2.50D and 2.50MA, respectively, as this condition is congruent. However, if one adds lenses or prisms, the stimulus demands are now unequal. For example, if one adds 6pd base-out, the accommodative stimulus remains 2.50D while the vergence stimulus becomes approximately 3.50MA.

CHAPTER 3
NEARWORK-INDUCED PERMANENT MYOPIA

HISTORICAL PERSPECTIVE

The association between one's near environment and myopia has been a long-standing controversy. This idea dates back to at least 1604, with Kepler being the first one credited with making this potentially important connection (Duke-Elder and Abrams 1970). He indicated that individuals engaged in considerable reading and writing became myopic (Goldschmidt 1968). Ramazzini (1713) also postulated that prolonged near activity resulted in changes in the "tonus of the membranes and fibers of the eye" which led to "weakness of vision." Similarly, Donders (1864) suggested that myopia occurred as a consequence of prolonged nearwork. More specifically, he attributed myopic development to "tension of the eyes for near objects."

In addition to Donders, other investigators proposed similar ideas. For example, upon observing the association between increased near visual activity and myopic onset, Cohn (1867, 1883) developed the classic "use-abuse theory." He postulated that myopia developed as a consequence of increased use of the eyes. More specifically, Cohn echoed similar nearwork-related myopigenic mechanisms as espoused by Donders. While this included convergence and the stooping position of the head, Cohn further postulated that accommodative effort caused elongation of the eye in genetically susceptible individuals, thus resulting in myopia.

The notion that nearwork is a primary factor in myopigenesis was a basic tenet of Skeffington, and later espoused by his proponents of the OEP viewpoint (see Birnbaum 1993 for a detailed review). In addition, other factors such as intrinsic task-related stress, cognitive function, and psychologic stress have been invoked (Forrest 1988). These ideas have added a degree of complexity to the potential factors contributing to the development of myopia.

An increased prevalence of myopia has been observed in certain groups associated with a greater level of education or in certain occupations involving intensive nearwork (Curtin 1985, Adams et al. 1989). The common element is nearwork. Goldschmidt (1968) stated that nearwork biases all refraction in the myopic direction. Duke-Elder (1949) summarized the relation of myopia and nearwork as follows: "Throughout all this maze of theorizing, much of it mutually contradictory and most of it fanciful, there run two main threads of thought linking the onset and progress of myopia with environmental constitutional factors—excessive close work and general debility." The above ideas are consistent with a recent medically-based statistical study clearly demonstrating the important role for environmental factors in the cause of myopia (Framingham Offspring Eye Study Group 1996).

SCHOOL MYOPIA

General School Population

Epidemiological surveys have consistently noted a higher prevalence of myopia in academically-based populations, with the former being related to the level of education (Baldwin et al. 1991). This was noted as early as 1813 (Ware). This association remained intact even after familial tendency towards myopia was taken into account (Wong et al. 1993). Myopia typically develops in children of school age and exhibits a gradual increase in prevalence, as well as in magnitude, from grade school through graduate school. Hence, the term "school myopia." The earliest data available implicating a causal relationship between educational level and myopia was reported by Cohn (1867, 1883). He investigated the refractive status of 10,060 schoolchildren in German cities and noted a trend towards increased myopia with age. While myopia occurred in approximately 5% of the children as early as in kindergarten, it increased to over 50% for students in professional and graduate schools. With his "use-abuse theory," Cohn (1867, 1883) postulated that the development of myopia served as an adaptive mechanism to meet the visual demands associated with near activity. The rationale was as follows: inherent in the educational process were reading and other close work which posed a "burden" on the eyes. This was responsible for triggering the onset of myopia, which effectively reduced the near accommodative demand.

The findings of Cohn (1867) were later confirmed by others. The earliest and oft-cited work in this area was conducted on Northern American natives. Morgan and Munro (1973) found a considerable increase in myopic prevalence for the younger generations who now attended school. This is particularly intriguing as significant refractive error had been a rare occurrence for Northern Eskimos and Indians until then. They reported that the prevalence peaked at 15-25 years of age, approaching a frequency as high as 35%. The prevalence exhibited a sharp decline on either end of this age range, with a frequency of ≤5% for ages ≤5 years or ≥25 years. Dietary changes and the process of "hybridization" were implicated as the most likely causes of the so-called myopia "epidemic." However, no evidence or additional data analyses were provided in support of these speculations. Furthermore, there was no age-matched control group.

A more definitive study was done by Richler and Bear (1980), who evaluated the relation between myopia, education, and nearwork habits of individuals from 3 separate rural communities in Newfoundland. The primary advantage of selecting this population was the natural minimization of racial influences due to their very limited migration and relatively homogeneous group composition. Non-cycloplegic refraction was performed on 957 individuals comprising approximately 80% of the population with ages ranging from 5-60 years. Information regarding education level and number of hours spent doing nearwork was also verbally obtained. The trends with age for refraction, duration of nearwork, and level of education exhibited a striking parallelism (Figure 3-1). Moderate but significant negative correlations (r = -0.26 to -0.49) was consistently reported between their refraction and amount of near work for all age groups, except those ≥60 years old. Refraction was consistently and significantly correlated with the amount of near work even after age, sex, and educational factors were taken into account. Likewise, poorer albeit significant negative correlations (r = -0.19 to -0.40) were found between refraction and educational level up to age 60 years. That is, increased myopia was found among those who performed a greater amount of nearwork, as well as among those who completed a greater number of years of education.

More recently, Sperduto et al. (1983) evaluated the prevalence of myopia as a function of several different parameters, including age and educational level. The study was based on a sample of 7,401 subjects aged 12-54 years obtained from the survey reports submitted by the National

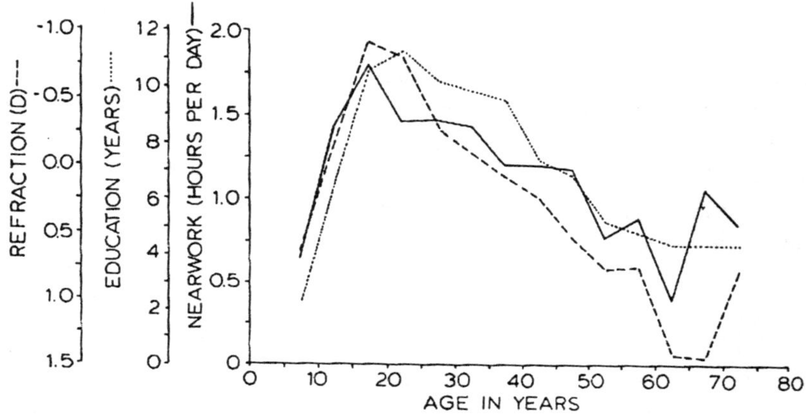

Figure 3-1 : Course of 5 year age group means of refraction, nearwork, and education (Reprinted with permission, Richler and Bear 1980).

Center for Health Statistics. Their analysis showed that the prevalence of myopia markedly increased with the highest grade of education completed. In fact, a significant difference in prevalence was reported between those completing less than 5 school years (3-6%) and those completing more than 12 school years (31%-40%). This difference in prevalence was independent of age.

In a more recent study of Jewish teenagers aged 14-18 years (Zylbermann et al. 1993), the prevalence and average degree of myopia were both noted to be significantly greater in orthodox males (81.3% and -2.90D, respectively) as compared to males from the general school population (27.4% and -0.50D, respectively) and to the female student population in both general (31.7% and -0.90D) and orthodox (36.2% and -0.90D) schools. No significant differences were found among the latter three groups. These notable differences between the orthodox male students and the other groups were believed to be related to the near demand inherent in the different school systems. General schools are coeducational and have similar programs, as in the typical Western school system. These programs only demand a moderate amount of near work. A typical school day lasts approximately six hours in length and is interspersed with hourly breaks. Homework does not exceed three hours per day. On the other hand, the orthodox schools offer a gender-specific curriculum. Programs in girls' orthodox schools are similar to those in general schools. In contrast, the curriculum offered in boys' orthodox schools is much more rigorous and is characterized by a substantial amount of sustained near vision, thus requiring longer and more sustained accommodation. It emphasizes the study of Jewish religious texts such as the Bible, the Talmud, etc., with the print size varying but frequently being of very small type, as little as 1 mm in height. The study hours increased considerably with age, from 3 hours per day for 4-year-olds to 16 hours per day for ages of 13 years and above. Reading is accompanied by frequent changes in the accommodative stimulus due to their to-and-fro swaying motion ("shukling"). This is probably one of the most convincing studies demonstrating the relation between amount of nearwork, and both the degree and the prevalence of myopia, as it has both homogeneous lifestyle and genetic components.

All of the above studies were cross-sectional in nature and by virtue of this, their validity may be somewhat limited due to individual variabilities across subjects. Therefore, to enable a subject to serve as his own control, a longitudinal study is more desirable. Such a study was undertaken by Duke-Elder (1930). Longitudinal examination of 244 students aged 14 to 20 years at the London School of Printing revealed a higher prevalence of myopia in subjects involved in courses requiring an extensive amount of near work. Compositors, whose task entailed the highest level of near work among all the students, exhibited a myopic prevalence of 42.5% upon initial examination. This was in contrast to those individuals engaged in less near work, e.g., warehousemen, who demonstrated a myopic prevalence of only 27%. Over a period of 3 years among the compositors, 16% of the emmetropes developed myopia, 77% of the original myopes continued to exhibit progression, and 31% of the hyperopes showed less hyperopia. Thus, a *refraction-independent myopic shift* was evident. On the other hand, among the warehousemen, none of the emmetropes became myopic, 33% of the initial myopes continued to progress, and 11.5% of the hyperopes became less hyperopic.

Another longitudinal study was conducted by Peckham et al. (1977) on younger age groups. A total of 11,179 children in the United Kingdom were examined at 7 and 11 years of age. Presenting data that were in support of other prevalence studies, myopia was reported to be more common among children of families engaged in non-manual labor versus those families engaged in manual labor, although the difference was not substantial (5% versus 3%). This is perhaps related to the fact that at these younger ages, myopia is still relatively infrequently found. In addition, they reported that the myopic children spent more of their leisure time reading. In fact, twice as many myopes versus other refractive groups indicated that they read during their spare time, and this was a statistically significant finding.

A recent study on an older population of 4533 Caucasian adults (aged 43 to 84 years) emphasized the relation between schoolwork and the degree of myopia (Wang et al. 1994). With the myopia criterion defined as a spherical correction greater than -0.50D, they concluded that an increased myopic prevalence was associated with the number of school years completed independent of age, as found in earlier studies. However, the relation was non-monotonic. Prevalence was greatest for those completing 12 years of school and decreased as the number of school years became greater or less than 12 years. On the other hand, mean magnitude of myopia was found to vary directly with the number of school years. It was greatest for subjects completing the highest number of school years regardless of age. However, including older subjects may have introduced undesirable extraneous factors. Refractive changes unrelated to nearwork in older presbyopic individuals are well documented (Slataper 1950, Hirsch 1958).

Graduate School Population

Since the occurrence of myopia was repeatedly demonstrated to be related to nearwork and its prevalence shown to increase with educational level, certain academically-oriented population groups who have completed a considerable amount of schooling or who are involved in intensive and excessive near visual activity due to demands of schoolwork, may therefore be more likely to exhibit myopia. An appropriate sample would be medical students, since they engage in a rigorous regimen of study over a number of years. One hundred and thirty-three medical university students (21-33 years) were examined using non-cycloplegic refraction (Midelfart et al. 1992). With myopia being defined as ≥-0.25 D (spherical equivalent), the prevalence was found to be 50%. This is a relatively high figure compared to the frequency obtained from the general population (~25%) (Sperduto et al. 1983). An even higher frequency was noted among optometry students (Septon 1984). Using a criterion of >-0.37D sph for myopia, the prevalence was 75%. These optometry students (n =500, 21-38 years of age) completed, on average, 5 years of post-secondary school education.

Further evidence has been provided by a longitudinal study covering a period of 2 years and consisting of a total of 3 annual cycloplegic refractions conducted on a randomly selected, young adult population (aged 20-30 years) from the Harvard Law and Business School (Dunphy et al. 1968). Approximately 60% of the sample (n =200) were initially myopic. Once again, this is a notably high figure compared to the prevalence of myopia in the general unselected population (~25%). An increase in the prevalence was evident even after only a year of graduate work, with half of the myopes becoming more myopic and a third of the non-myopes shifting in the myopic direction. Once again, a general myopic shift was evident. This myopic shift in law students was also reported by Zadnik and Mutti (1987).

More recently, a cohort investigation of the myopic prevalence of medical students aged 18-21 years at the National Taiwan University was documented (Lin et al. 1996). The prevalence of myopia at the commencement of the study was approximately 93%, which was considerably higher than that reported by any other investigation. Over a period of 5 years, the myopic prevalence in these students increased by 3% resulting in approximately 96%. This 3% increase can be attributed to the development of late-onset myopia in the small group (7%) of initially emmetropic individuals. The mean increase in myopia was 0.68D. This was accounted for by a significant increase in axial length (mean change of 0.49mm), according to the authors. None of the other ocular components, including corneal radius, anterior chamber depth, and lens thickness manifested any significant changes over this same period.

Military Academic Population

An increased prevalence of myopia also seemed to characterize students attending the military academy. Rosner and Belkin (1987) conducted a nationwide study of young Israeli male military recruits (n = 157,748) aged 17-19 years. Thus, this study had the advantage of controlling for possible age effects. Information regarding the educational level of each subject was obtained. Data analysis revealed a strong correlation between myopia and years of schooling. Prevalence of myopia for those completing 8 years or less of schooling was 7.5%. This increased slightly as the number of school years increased, followed by a significantly and markedly higher value of 19.7% for those completing 12 school years or more, thus exhibiting an increase of over 2.5 times in the most highly educated.

Similar refractive shifts were also reported among other studies of military recruits as the development and progression of ametropia were documented through most of their education at the military academy (Sutton and Ditmars 1970). Entering freshman cadets from five classes (1968-1972) at the US Military Academy had an ametropic prevalence of 47.5%, which increased to 62.2% upon graduation. Unfortunately, the criterion used was a requirement to wear corrective spectacles, and therefore it was not clear whether all the reported cases consisted solely of myopes, although this was probably true of most.

A study by Paritsis et al. (1983) conducted on 474 military servicemen found that the group who had completed over 10 years of schooling had three times more myopia than the group who completed less than 10 years of schooling. According to the authors, when this factor was coupled with the amount of time spent in an urban environment, it was related to the *onset* rather than the progression of myopia.

A longitudinal, retrospective study of 497 cadets aged 17-21 years was conducted at the United States Air Force Academy (O'Neal and Connon 1987). Myopic frequency was 44.2% for entering cadets. During the course of the first 2.5 years, this frequency increased to 53.7%. 48% of the initial hyperopes, 41% of the initial emmetropes, and 74% of the initial myopes developed changes in the myopic direction (Figure 3-2), suggesting once again an overall general "myopization" trend rather than simply the case of emmetropes now becoming late-onset myopes. Their data indicated that eyes with higher refractive errors exhibited greater myopic shifts.

Myopic shifts were also observed among midshipmen after admission to the United States Naval Academy (Hayden 1941). Hayden reported that the frequency of those who developed "defective" vision ranged from 14 to 32% during the course of their studies. The vast majority of individuals who were initially emmetropic or hyperopic were found to develop approximately 0.50D of myopia within one to four years after admission to the academy. This refractive shift was, according to Hayden, the result of intensive studying. Thus, to remain qualified for commission after completion of four years at the academy, Hayden recommended that a 1D hyperopic buffer be instituted for all admitted candidates. Clearly, this is consistent with attempts to prevent occurrence of such myopia using plus lenses for near, accommodative rock exercises, and more frequent rest periods with

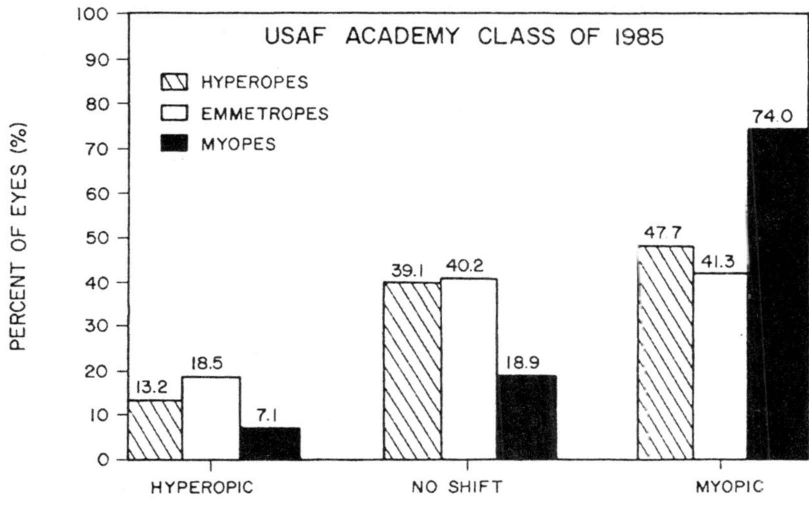

Figure 3-2 : Percentage of eyes in each type of entering SPEQ (spherical equivalent) refractive error showing a hyperopic or myopic shift of ≤0.25D or no shift (≤0.12D) in SPEQ between the entrance and third academic year examinations (2.5 year period) for 994 eyes from USAFA class of 1985 (Reprinted with permission, O'Neal and Connon 1987).

distant viewing, as the impact on the individual and cost to society are considerable.

A study by Teasdale and colleagues (1988) looked at the relation between myopic prevalence/ progression and educational attainment. An investigation of 15,834 18-year-old Danish military draftees showed that a third of this population was myopic, with a range from -0.25D to -7.75D, while the remaining two-thirds were emmetropic. Similar to previous findings, the prevalence of myopia appeared to increase in proportion to educational level. A significant increase from 7 to 30% was noted as the educational level increased from 8 to 13 years. The mean educational level attained for myopes was significantly greater than for the emmetropes. Furthermore, low myopes (myopia of less than 2 D) had significantly less years of education than moderate and high myopes (myopia exceeding 2 D). However, the degree of myopia and educational level were not correlated for myopias greater than 2 D. It was further concluded that the factor associated with education determined the onset of myopia, but played less of a role in determining the degree of myopic progression, as was also suggested by Paritsis et al. (1983).

The Role of Schoolwork in Myopia—Precursor or Consequence?

Does near work induce myopia or are myopes more inclined to engage in near tasks, either due to their initially limiting uncorrected ametropia or due to other factors such as their personality? It has been widely held that myopic children gravitated towards more scholarly activities (Duke-Elder 1949), that they were more academically-inclined, or simply more comfortable in the engagement of nearwork. This was rationalized to be related to their poor uncorrected distant vision which compromised their ability to pursue active physical activities such as sports, thereby compelling them to spend more time performing sedentary tasks (Borish 1970). However, this notion was refuted by Young (1971). He argued that it is relatively uncommon for ametropic children to function with unaided vision, especially when the corrected vision was just as good as the habitual vision of emmetropes. In addition, Peckham et al. (1977) noted that both myopes and non-myopes participated in outdoor sports to a similar degree. Furthermore, Paritsis et al. (1983) reported that the same percentage of subjects (75%) who belonged to groups differentiated by their frequency of myopia exhibited a similar inclination towards studying. Additionally, based on his years of clinical experience, Birnbaum (1993) indicated that interest in reading usually *preceded* the development of myopia. Similarly, intellectual gain *precedes* the development of myopia in children (Karlsson, 1975; Peckham et al, 1977; Sofaer and Emery, 1981). Finally, the phenomenon of late-onset myopia (see later discussion in this chapter) implicates the role of environment in the etiology of myopia. Therefore, from the evidence presented so far, it appears that *nearwork plays a prominent role in the development of myopia, at least in certain subgroups.*

OCCUPATIONAL MYOPIA

Myopia had also long been observed to occur with a higher frequency in certain occupational groups. The term "occupational myopia" was thus derived from the relation between these groups and their myopia. A review of the literature reveals that nearly a century of studies in this area has yielded remarkably similar results. Table 3-1 compares data collected from several of these studies. Occupational categories were based on the estimated amount of near work involved. A duplication of Tscherning's (1882, 1920) study by Goldschmidt (1968) using the same occupational categories produced strikingly similar results. In a given population at a specific time, the prevalence of myopia was reported to be greatest for those who were involved in a substantial amount of near work or engaged in sustained fine near tasks, as would be true of students or writers, as opposed to seamen and laborers who were at the other end of the spectrum and presented with the least amount of near work and overall substantially less near visual demands (Table 3-1).

TABLE 3-1: RELATIVE FREQUENCY OF MYOPIA IN VARIOUS OCCUPATIONAL GROUPS

	Professionals, Writers, Students	Musicians, Engineers	Carpenters, Bakers, Workmen	Farmers, Seamen, Laborers
Tscherning (1882)	32%	13%	5%	2%
Seggel (1884)	57%		9%	2%
Duke-Elder (1930)	43%			
Giles (1950)	36%			21%
Goldschmidt (1968)	39%	20%	9%	6%

The frequency of myopia was determined on a group of individuals who primarily performed either near or far tasks (Nyman 1988). Near task workers consisted of VDT operators, typists, word processors, map drawers, etc. Far task workers consisted of policemen. An increased frequency of myopia was reported for those who perform near versus far work in the younger age groups. However, according to the study, this does not implicate nearwork in the causation of myopia. This increased frequency was attributed to natural selection. Given the common nature of VDT's and word processing in both the workplace and home, however, it seems that "natural selection" could not be the sole factor.

Another investigation of a longitudinal nature was conducted by Tokoro (1988) on a sample of 528 subjects aged 20-59 years. Non-cycloplegic refraction with an autorefractor was assessed before and after one year of VDT work. A small (0.09-0.14D) but statistically significant increase in myopia was found for the younger age groups (20-39 years). No change in myopia was found for the older age groups (>40 years), presumably because they had little if any residual accommodation. A significant correlation was found between myopic change and time engaged in near work for the 30-39 year-old group. However, no control group was evaluated to determine if any of these changes were in fact the consequence of VDT usage or simply occurred in a subgroup of individuals as a natural process.

The most-cited contemporary work in this area is probably that of Adams and McBrien (1992b), who determined the prevalence of myopia and myopic progression in a population of clinical binocular microscopists. A total of 251 subjects were used with a mean age of approximately 30 years. The distribution of refractive errors was determined using non-cycloplegic refraction. 6% of the total number of 502 eyes were hyperopic (>+0.75 D), 28% were emmetropic (-0.25 to +0.75 D), and an overwhelming 66% were myopic (≥-0.375D). The authors also indicated that this prevalence of myopia was almost twice as much as that found in other studies (37%) for unselected population samples of similar ages. However, there was no relation between myopic change and the amount of time spent doing near tasks either at or outside of work, perhaps suggesting a saturation phenomenon, even when a comparison was made between the subgroup who reported at least one prescription change following entry into the profession and the remaining subgroup which did not. The only significant difference between these two groups was their ages, with the former group having a mean age of 31 years and the latter group having a mean age of 27 years. The results suggest that near work may be related to the *onset* of myopic progression, but neither to the total amount of myopia nor its rate of progression. Thus, as found in studies discussed earlier, *nearwork seems to act as a trigger mechanism for its development of myopia, in particular the onset.* The authors attributed their findings to factors present in this special type of occupational task. See later discussion with respect to their myopic progression.

Further evidence for occupational myopia was provided by Tatevosyan (1968). He reported that unilateral myopia developed in the viewing eye of approximately 28% of the females engaged in monocular microscopy.

DOES GENETICS OR ENVIRONMENT PLAY A MORE DOMINANT ROLE IN INDUCING MYOPIA?

Few studies have been conducted with the specific purpose of delineating the role of heredity versus environment in the pathogenesis of myopia. In an attempt by Young et al. (1969) to minimize genetic variations and isolate environmental factors, a cross-sectional study of individuals of the same ethnic origin was conducted. The transmission of refractive errors within Eskimo families was investigated. Cycloplegic refraction was performed on a total 508 Eskimos ranging in age from 6-77 years. Data analyzed with reference to age showed that the prevalence of myopia in those over 40 years was disproportionately low. It approximated 2%, which was a considerably and significantly smaller percentage than the 45% found for the younger individuals (<40 years). In addition, a comparative study of

3 generations within the same family unit was done. There was no evidence of myopia in the grandparents. They were hyperopic, ranging from +0.25 D to +6.44 D. Only 8% of the parents were myopic, while 60% of the third generation schoolchildren were myopic. Thus, there was a large and consistent generational myopic increase. The mean refraction for the parents was +1.69 ± 1.55 D (SD) as compared to +0.33 ± 2.37 D (SD) in the children.

In this study, heredity could not have been a major variable. If this were so, the majority of children would not exhibit myopia, since their parents and/or grandparents were predominantly hyperopic. The authors suggested that the relatively sudden increase in prevalence and the greater degree of myopia in the younger generation may be related to external influences. They noted that this dramatic increase in myopia in the younger generations coincided with the introduction of Western influences, with particular emphasis on compulsory schooling for them. The parents were illiterate, while their children were formally educated for many years in schools. To prove their point further, data from 41 family units were separately analyzed. Correlation between members of the same family were performed. No significant correlations were found for parent-child refractions, but intersibling correlations were found. Thus, the authors concluded that the difference in findings could not be due to heredity. Rather they suggested that the environment, i.e., common familial environmental factors, now played a dominant role. However, they acknowledged the possibility that the attitudes of parents toward education may have also played an important part. The authors then partialed out age effects statistically, since some young children were used whose refractive status may not yet have stabilized, and hence might influence the correlation. Essentially the same result was again found.

More recently, Mohan et al. (1988) conducted a study using relatively young patients (200 individuals, 10-21 years of age) selected from a clinical population. To accomplish their aim of evaluating the relative role of genetics versus environment, the subjects were interviewed regarding their daily average amount of near work, with near work being defined as any task performed at a distance of 50 cm or less. Information was also obtained regarding their family history of refraction. Subjects were then divided into myopes and non-myopes based on their cycloplegic refraction. They were further subdivided with regard to the presence of a family history of myopia. The results revealed that over three times more myopes than non-myopes were involved in 6 hours or more of near work per day, i.e., about 70% of the myopes as compared to 20% of the non-myopes. The average number of hours spent performing nearwork per day was 4-5 for the non-myopes, which was statistically different from the 6-9 reported by the myopes. Interestingly, the myopic group without a family history of myopia did the most near work. These findings argue in favor of the predominant role of the environment in the development of myopia. It also takes credence away from the alternative explanations advanced by proponents of the genetics theory, which suggested that predisposition to myopia was primarily genetically-determined (Goldschmidt 1968).

Nonetheless, the effect of heredity cannot be totally discounted. Its role is evidenced in the increased degree of concordance of refraction in uniovular twins, even with different geographical conditions (Young 1977). Moreover, not everyone subjected to nearwork will exhibit a myopic increase. Some individuals may be more susceptible to nearwork-related factors than others. It will be important in future studies to determine those history-related factors and clinical findings that may predispose an individual to become myopic (see Chapter 7). With such information, more effective preventive measures can be developed.

Perhaps the role of heredity and environment in the development of myopia can be better delineated if we can appreciate the fact that there are two primary etiologies in the development of myopia, each of which can occur independently or co-exist with the manifest myopia being the sum total. The inherited myopic component is believed to develop primarily during early childhood concurrent with the period of maximal physical growth, while the environmentally-induced myopia is found in persons involved in performing substantial amount of nearwork, with its onset believed to occur primarily later in life after the cessation of bodily growth (Goldschmidt 1968). However, there may be a genetic predisposition or susceptibility. And, these two components may occur concurrently to differing degrees. What mechanisms are responsible for the myopia? A growing body of evidence suggests a final axial contribution, although the lens mechanism and related retinal defocus may be a predisposing factor in specific subgroups (Ong and Ciuffreda, 1995). See Chapters 4-6 for further discussion of this important topic.

LATE-ONSET MYOPIA

The influence of one's environment on myopia, particularly in younger age groups, is frequently obscured by the normal pattern of ocular growth. Therefore, it may be helpful to look at refractive changes occurring in individuals past their expected normal general and ocular growth developmental stages. The classical concept with regard to myopic progression was that it stabilized during the late teens or early adulthood (Goss and Winkler 1983). This was largely based on longitudinal studies involving the developmental changes in the ocular refractive components (Sorsby et al. 1961), which showed that ocular growth was completed at approximately 15 years of age, with this occurring somewhat earlier in females than males (Goss 1991). However, changing visual demands, biasing of work in enclosed or near environments (Septon 1984), and increasing emphasis on higher education compel us to rethink and perhaps modify these traditional views. More recent cross-sectional as well as longitudinal studies, particularly those on academic and occupational groups characterized by extensive near work as discussed earlier, demonstrate a susceptibility to the onset and to a lesser extent the progression of myopia well beyond the traditional developmental years in a substantial subgroup of individuals. Goldschmidt (1968) distinguished this type of myopic development that occurred after the cessation of physical growth as "spatmyopie," e.g., of a spasm nature. He also believed that it was environmental in origin and not likely to be genetically-induced. Goss and Winkler (1983) and Grosvenor (1987), among others, have classified this type of myopia as "late-onset myopia or early adult-onset myopia". Lindner (1949) suggested that it may be axial in nature. On the other hand, Goldschmidt (1968) and Sato (1957) speculated that it was lenticular in origin.

Interestingly, in a recent study by Midelfart et al. (1992) as discussed earlier in this chapter, the prevalence of myopia among a group of medical students was 50%. When queried as to when they received their first pair of corrective lenses, the mean reported age was 16 years (range 7-23 years) with 43% of the myopes having an onset occurring at or *after* 19 years of age. Thus, approximately 25% of the original sample appear to be late-onset myopes. According to the authors, the myopia was presumed to be related to an excessive near demand from reading, which produced a "stress" of the accommodative mechanism, thereby leading to myopia.

A potentially interesting resource group for studying late-onset myopia is found among military draftees. (See earlier sections on military academy and graduate school populations.) Studies conducted at military academies have provided strong evidence for the late environmental role in myopia. Due to the stringent visual standards set by the academy, the entire entering class typically consists of non-myopes, generally 17-21 years of age. Therefore, any myopia developing following the commencement of their studies will clearly have an onset past the developmental years, i.e., late-onset myopia. One such report was conducted at the United States Naval Academy (Hynes 1956). Refraction was obtained for the same class upon entry and then four years later upon graduation. A *relative* myopic refractive shift occurred across all ages. An increased likelihood to develop myopia was found for the younger as well as the less hyperopic individuals. Approximately 85% of the youngest entering age group (17-18 year-olds) developed myopia over the course of four years, while less than 20% of the oldest age group (21 year-olds) did, thus suggesting greater susceptibility in the younger individuals. In addition, individuals with an initial cycloplegic refraction of ≤+0.50D demonstrated a considerably greater myopic frequency upon graduation regardless of their age. For the youngest age group, 70% of those with an initial refraction of ≤+0.50D developed myopia as compared with less than 5% of the initial hyperopes with refractive errors ≥+1.00D. For the oldest age group, 10% of those with an initial refraction of ≤+0.50D developed myopia versus 5% of those whose initial refraction was ≥+1.00D. Further analysis of the data revealed that a myopic shift in refraction occurred across all refractive groups. Sixty-seven percent of the initial hyperopes of at least 1D became less hyperopic, while the number of individuals with a refraction of ≤+0.50D increased sevenfold over this span of time. These results provide potent evidence that *all* refractive groups were susceptible to environmental influences and showed a general myopic trend, as discussed earlier in this chapter.

Simensen and Thorud (1994) compared the refraction of textile workers to a control group matched in terms of age, sex, and educational level. The experimental group was involved in near textile work (working distance= 30 cm) for an average of 16 years, while the control group consisted of clerical and sales-related activities in the same factory. Statistically significant differences in the cycloplegic refraction were found, with the control group showing a mean of +1.19D and the experimental group mean of -2.56D. A significant difference in axial length of 1.66mm was also found suggesting that the eventual myopic difference was primarily of an axial nature. Ninety-one percent of the near workers were myopic, with 80% of them acquiring myopia at least 6 months *after* they commenced work at the textile factory. All of the experimental workers appeared to be late-onset myopes, with their myopia being diagnosed at or after 17 years of age. None of the control workers were myopic. In addition, the magnitude of myopia was found to increase with the number of years spent in the trade. However, some potential problems with the study need to be addressed. First, it involved a relatively small sample of subjects (n =22). Secondly, some incomplete information makes comparison somewhat difficult.

In another recent investigation of a longitudinal nature as mentioned earlier in this chapter, Adams and McBrien (1992b) reported that 71% of a population of clinical microscopists were myopic in at least one eye. Of the total population sample, approximately one-half reported at least one prescription change due to increased myopia after entry into this field. Of the latter group, approximately 50% reported an initial onset of myopia occurring *after* becoming a microscopist at a median age of 26 years. Another interesting and important finding was that the majority of subjects reported a progression of their myopia *after* entry into their profession in the *absence* of any myopic changes having occurred in the 5 years preceding their entry at age 16-17 years, with this being the age during which most myopia is reported to cease developing (Goss and Winkler 1983). It appeared that the myopia stabilized for a considerable period of time, after which a renewal of myopic progression occurred which correlated closely with entry into their profession. The authors attributed their findings to the near occupational task. Thus, once again markedly increased nearwork appeared to act as a trigger mechanism for myopic development. It should be emphasized, however, that a differential susceptibility to such an environmental stimulus appears to exist, since not everyone engaged in this same profession developed myopia.

The prevalence of late-onset myopia appears to be approximately 10% in the general population (Grosvenor 1987, O'Neal and Connon 1987), which represents roughly one-third of the 25-30% myopic prevalence in the general population (Sperduto et al. 1983, Grosvenor 1987). In special populations involved in substantial nearwork activity, the prevalence was similar (O'Neal and Connon 1987, Adams and McBrien 1992b, Midelfart et al. 1992, Simensen and Thorud 1994). Thus, late-onset myopia is a relatively common refractive condition that deserves further investigation, especially in light of increasing daily nearwork demands in our society. Clinical trials to understand more precisely its epidemiology, predisposing factors, susceptibility, and possible preventive measures are needed in this important clinical condition.

EXPERIMENTAL ANIMAL DATA

Although the animal results have clearly demonstrated the striking effect that one's environment has on refractive development, the impact of near vision on refractive error can better be appreciated and made more relevant by selecting or manipulating the visual environment such that vision is restricted to specific distances only. Barrett (1932) found differences in refraction between domesticated and wild animals. While myopia was reported among the domesticated animals, it was not found in any of the wild animals. Likewise, a sample of caged cats confined in rooms with dimensions measuring 2 x 2 x 3.3m were found to be predominantly myopic (75.8%) as compared to a control group of nondomesticated street cats which were predominantly (87.5%) hyperopic (Belkin et al. 1977). Once again, this implicates the near visual environment in myopigenesis, although the ensuing myopia in this case was *not* axial in nature (Rose et al. 1974, Belkin et al. 1977). In addition, Young (1964) reported that similarly aged rhesus monkeys reared in the wilderness versus in the laboratory yielded different mean refractive errors. Wild rhesus monkeys had a mean refractive error of +0.63D, which was significantly different from the mean refractive error of +0.06D exhibited by the laboratory-reared rhesus monkeys. Further analysis of the data obtained from the monkey population was performed by Young (1967), which was then compared to human data obtained from two independent studies. These studies included the Pullman study (Young et al. 1954) which comprised a reading population, and the Washington study (Kempf et al. 1928) which used a non-reading population. Again, there was a link between nearwork and myopia.

Artificial restriction of the visual environment to no more than a few inches was also successful in inducing myopia. Work on neonate chicks (Wallman et al. 1978, 1981) showed that these animals developed severe myopia (a mean of -10D and a median of -22D) when vision was restricted to the frontal field of view. Corresponding increases in the vitreous chamber, axial length, and corneal curvature were also noted. Vision confined to the lateral field of view yielded a mean refractive error of +1.9D with no change in axial length. This was not surprising. Since the lateral fields, which are used for distance vision, were essentially eliminated in the frontal-field birds, vision was then confined only to near, thus once again supporting the role of near vision in myopic development. It was further indicated in the study that accommodation appeared to be responsible for the myopization process, since sectioning of the ciliary nerve reduced the myopia by a considerable amount (median value of only -4D). Furthermore, the mechanism by which the loss of accommodation hindered myopic development was attributed to its effect on corneal curvature. It was argued that in birds, contraction of the ciliary muscle exert centripetal force on the corneal margin, thereby reducing its radius. This, of course, is not true in humans.

Myopia was also successfully demonstrated in laboratory-induced near environments (Young 1961a,b). Eighteen macaques were used, ranging in age from 4 to 6 years (Young 1961b), which was approximately equivalent to humans aged 11-17 years (Young 1964). Half of the macaques were in the experimental group and confined to restraining chairs which were enclosed in hoods that restricted vision to within 20 inches (Figure 3-3). In contrast, the remaining half of the monkeys which served as controls were reared in cages placed in a large room. All monkeys remained in their respective environments for at least 4 months. Cycloplegic refraction following 8 months of confinement revealed that both groups of monkeys became more myopic. The experimental group exhibited 0.75 D more myopia, while the control group had an increase of only 0.19 D. The relatively consistent effect obtained in these two groups of monkeys despite a random hereditary background suggested that the environment played a crucial role in their myopic development. Subsequent investigations likewise produced similar results (Young 1962, 1963, 1964, 1965, 1967, 1977).

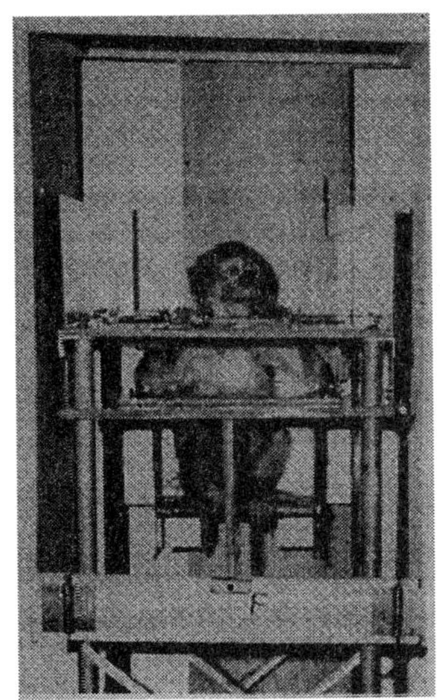

Figure 3-3 : Monkey named Elliven sitting in a restraining chair in the hood (Reprinted with permission, Young 1961b).

While investigations involving animals have provided evidence in support of the relation between nearwork and myopia, nonetheless, some caution should be practiced when applying animal findings to humans (Edwards 1996). The visual system between humans and animals is undeniably different (Zadnik and Mutti 1995). Even within the primate group, there are species differences which may yield different results (Raviola and Wiesel 1980, 1985, 1990). Clearly, more investigations involving large-scale clinical trials in humans are needed.

SUMMARY

The association between nearwork and the development of myopia in both humans and animals has been well documented in the literature. In numerous human studies, the level of one's educational attainment or the nature of one's occupation were used as indices of the degree of nearwork activity. In addition, several of these studies also showed that nearwork was primarily related to the onset rather than the progression of myopia. And, recent studies in late-onset myopes more firmly establish the role of nearwork as a primary etiological factor.

REFERENCES

Adams AJ, Baldwin WR, Biederman I, Curtin BJ, Ebenholtz SM, Goss DA, Hutchison GB, Seddon JM, Wallman J. Myopia-prevalence and progression. Washington, DC: National Academy Press; 1989.

Adams DW, McBrien NA. Prevalence of myopia and myopic progression in a population of clinical microscopists. Optom Vis Sci. 1992b; 69: 467-73.

Baldwin WR. Clinical research and procedures in refraction. In: Hirsch MJ, ed. Synopsis of the refractive state of the eye, a symposium. Minneapolis: Burgess; 1967: 39-59.

Baldwin WR, Adams AJ, Flattau P. Young-adult myopia. In: Grosvenor T, Flom MC, eds. Refractive anomalies- research and clinical applications. Boston: Butterworth-Heinemann; 1991: 104-20.

Barrett JW. The causation of myopia. Br J Ophthalmol. 1932; 16: 764-5.

Belkin M, Yinon U, Rose L, Reisert I. Effect of visual environment on refractive error of cats. Doc Ophthalmol. 1977; 42: 433-7.

Birnbaum MH. Optometric management of nearpoint vision disorders. Boston: Butterworth-Heinemann; 1993.

Borish IM. Clinical refraction, 3rd ed. Chicago: Professional Press Inc.; 1970.

Cohn H. Untersuchungen der augen von 10,060 schulkindern, nebst vorschlagen zur verbesserung der den augen nachteiligen schulemichtungen. Leipzig: Verlag von Freidrich Fleischer, 1867. Cited in Golschmidt E. On the etiology of myopia-an epidemiological study. Acta Ophthalmol (Suppl). 1968; 98: 1-171.

Cohn H. Hygiene of the eye in schools. Turnbull WP, ed. London: Simpkin, Marshall and Co.; 1883.

Curtin BJ. The etiology of myopia. In: The myopias: basic science and clinical management. Philadelphia: Harper and Row; 1985: 61-151.

Donders FC. On the anomalies of accommodation and refraction of the eye. trans. Moore WD. London: The New Sydenham Society; 1864.

Duke-Elder WS. An investigation into the effect upon the eyes of occupations involving close work. Br J Ophthalmol. 1930; 14: 609-20.

Duke-Elder WS. Textbook of ophthalmology, Vol. 4. London: C.V. Mosby Co.; 1949: 4243-413.

Duke-Elder S, Abrams D. System of ophthalmology, Vol. 5. Ophthalmic Optics and Refraction. London: Henry Kimpton; 1970.

Dunphy EB, Stoll MR, King SH. Myopia among American male graduate students. Am J Ophthalmol. 1968; 65: 518-21.

Edwards MH. Animal models of myopia. Acta Ophthalmol Scand. 1996; 74: 213-9.

Forrest EB. Stress and vision. Santa Ana: OEP Foundation; 1988.

Framingham Offspring Eye Study Group. Familial aggregation and prevalence of myopia in the Framingham Offspring Eye Study. Arch Ophthalmol. 1996: 114: 326-32.

Goldschmidt E. On the etiology of myopia-an epidemiological study. Copenhagen: Munksgaard. Acta Ophthalmol (Suppl). 1968; 98: 1-172.

Goss DA. Childhood myopia. In: Grosvenor T, Flom MC, eds. Refractive anomalies-research and clinical applications. Boston: Butterworth-Heinemann; 1991: 81-103.

Goss DA, Winkler RL. Progression of myopia in youth: age of cessation. Am J Optom Physiol Opt. 1983; 60: 651-8.

Grosvenor T. A review and a suggested classification system for myopia on the basis of age-related prevalence and age of onset. Am J Optom Physiol Opt. 1987; 64: 545-54.

Grosvenor T. Myopia and its development. In: Primary care optometry. New York: Professional Press Books/Fairchild Publications; 1989: 57-89.

Hayden R. Development and prevention of myopia at the United States Naval Academy. Arch Ophthalmol. 1941; 25: 539-47.

Hirsch MJ. Changes in refractive state after the age of 45. Am J Optom Arch Am Acad Optom. 1958; 35: 229-37.

Hynes EA. Refractive changes in normal young men. Arch Ophthalmol. 1956; 56: 761-7.

Karlsson JL. Influence of the myopia gene on brain development. Clin Genet. 1975;8:314-8.

Kempf GA, Collins SD, Jarman BL. Refractive errors in the eyes of children as determined by retinoscopic examination with a cycloplegic. Public Health Bulletin. Washington: US Gov Printing Office; 1928: 182.

Lin LLK, Shih YF, Lee YC, Hung PT, Hou PK. Changes in ocular refraction and its components among medical students- a 5-year longitudinal study. Optom Vis Sci. 1996; 73: 495-8.

Lindner K. Gedanken über den Vorgang der myopischen Dehnung und seine Hintanhaltung. Albrecht v. Graefes Arch Ophthalmol. 1949; 149: 293-317. Cited in Goldschmidt E. On the etiology of myopia-an epidemiological study. Acta Ophthalmol (Suppl). 1968; 98: 1-171.

Midelfart AM, Aamo B, Sjohaug KA, Dysthe BE. Myopia among medical students in Norway. Acta Ophthalmol. 1992; 70: 317-22.

Mohan M, Pakrasi S, Garg SP. The role of environmental factors and hereditary predisposition in the causation of low myopia. Acta Ophthalmol (Suppl). 1988; 185: 54-7.
Morgan RW, Munro M. Refractive problems in northern natives. Can J Ophthalmol. 1973; 8: 226-8.
Nyman KG. Occupational near-work myopia. Acta Ophthalmol (Suppl). 1988; 185: 167-71.
O'Neal MR, Connon TR. Refractive error change at the United States Air Force Academy-class of 1985. Am J Optom Physiol Opt.1987; 64: 344-54.
Ong E, Ciuffreda KJ. Nearwork-induced transient myopia-a critical review. Doc Ophthalmol. 1995; 91: 57-85.
Paritsis N, Sarafidou E, Koliopoulos J, Trichopoulos D. Epidemiologic research on the role of studying and urban environment in the development of myopia during school-age years. Annals Ophthalmol. 1983; 15: 1061-5.
Peckham CS, Gardiner PA, Goldstein H. Acquired myopia in 11-year-old children. Br Med J. 1977; 1: 542-5.
Ramazzini B. Diseases of workers. trans Wright WC. Chicago: University of Chicago Press; 1713. Cited in Owens DA, Wolf-Kelly K. Near work, visual fatigue and variations of oculomotor tonus. Invest Ophthalmol Vis Sci. 1987; 28: 743-9.
Raviola E, Wiesel TN. Effects of atropine on experimental myopia in macaque monkeys. Invest Ophthalmol Vis Sci (Suppl). 1980; 170-1.
Raviola E, Wiesel TN. An animal model of myopia. New Engl J Med. 1985; 312: 1609-15.
Raviola E, Wiesel TN. Neural control of eye growth and experimental myopia in primates. In: Myopia and the Control of Eye Growth-Ciba Foundation Symposium. Chichester: John Wiley & Sons; 1990: 22-44.
Richler A, Bear JC: Refraction, nearwork and education-a population study in Newfoundland. Acta Ophthalmol. 58: 468-78, 1980.
Rose L, Yinon U, Belkin M. Myopia induced in cats deprived of distance vision during development. Vis Res. 1974; 14: 1029-32.
Rosner M, Belkin M. Intelligence, education and myopia in males. Arch Ophthalmol. 1987; 105: 1508-11.
Sato T. The causes and prevention of acquired myopia. Yokohama: Helarudo Printing Co. Ltd.; 1957.
Septon RD. Myopia among optometry students. Am J Optom Physiol Opt. 1984; 61: 745-51.
Shapiro A, Stollman EB, Merin S. Do sex, ethnic origin or environment affect myopia? Acta Ophthalmol. 1982; 60: 803-8.
Simensen B, Thorud LO. Adult-onset myopia and occupation. Acta Ophthalmol. 1994; 72: 469-71.
Slataper FJ. Age norms of refraction and vision. Arch Ophthalmol. 1950; 43: 466-81.
Sofaer JA, Emery AEH. Genes for super-intelligence? J Med Genet. 1981;18:410-3.
Sorsby A, Benjamin B, Sheridan M. Refraction and its components during the growth of the eye from the age of three. Med Res Council Special Report Series no. 301. London: Her Majesty's Stationery Office; 1961.
Sperduto RD, Seigel D, Roberts J, Rowland M. Prevalence of myopia in the United States. Arch Ophthalmol. 1983; 101: 405-7.
Sutton MR, Ditmars DL. Vision problems at West Point. J Am Optom Assoc. 1970; 41: 263-5.
Teasdale TW, Fuchs J, Goldschmidt E. Degree of myopia in relation to intelligence and educational level. Lancet. 1988: 2; 1351-4.
Tokoro T. Effect of visual display terminal (VDT) work on myopia progression. Acta Ophthalmol (Suppl). 1988; 185: 172-4.

Tscherning M. Studier over myopiens ætiologi. Kobenhavn; 1882: 29-97. Cited in Goldschmidt E. On the etiology of myopia- an epidemiological study. Acta Ophthalmol (Suppl). 1968; 98: 1-171.

Tscherning M. Physiologic Optics, 3rd ed. trans Weiland C. Philadelphia: The Keystone Publishing Co.; 1920: 102.

Wallman J, Rosenthal D, Adams JI, Trachtman JN, Romagnano L. Role of accommodation and developmental aspects of experimental myopia in chicks. In: Fledelius HC, Alsbirk PH, Goldschmidt E, eds. Third International Conference on Myopia, Copenhagen. The Hague: Dr W. Junk Publishers. Doc Ophthalmol Proc Series. 1981; 28: 197-206.

Wallman J, Turkel J, Trachtman J. Extreme myopia produced by modest change in early visual experience. Science. 1978; 201: 1249-51.

Wang Q, Klein BEK, Klein R, Moss SE. Refractive status in the Beaver Dam eye study. Invest Ophthalmol Vis Sci. 1994; 35: 4344-7.

Ware J. Observations relative to the near and distant sight of different persons. Phil Trans R Soc Lond. 1813; 1: 31.

Wong L, Coggon D, Cruddas M, Hwang CH. Education, reading, and familial tendency as risk factors for myopia in Hong Kong fishermen. J Epidemiol Comm Health. 1993; 47: 50-3.

Young FA. The development and retention of myopia by monkeys. Am J Optom Arch Am Acad Optom. 1961a; 38: 545-55.

Young FA. The effect of restricted visual space on the primate eye. Am J Ophthalmol. 1961b; 52: 799-806.

Young FA. The effect of nearwork illumination level on monkey refraction. Am J Optom Arch Am Acad Optom. 1962; 39: 60-7.

Young FA. The effect of restricted visual space on the refractive error of the young monkey eye. Invest Ophthalmol. 1963; 2: 571-7.

Young FA. The distribution of refractive errors in monkeys. Exp Eye Res. 1964; 3: 230-8.

Young FA. The effect of atropine on the development of myopia in monkeys. Am J Optom Arch Am Acad Optom. 1965; 42: 439-49.

Young FA. Animal experimentation and research on refractive state. In: Hirsch MJ, ed. Synopsis of the refractive state of the eye-a symposium. Amer Acad Optom Series, Minneapolis:Burgess. 1967; 5: 26-38.

Young FA. The development of myopia. Contacto. 1971; 15: 36-42.

Young FA. The nature and control of myopia. J Am Optom Assoc. 1977; 48: 451-7.

Young FA, Beattie RJ, Newby FJ, Swindal MT. The Pullman study-a visual survey of Pullman school children- part II. Am J Optom. 1954; 31: 192-203.

Young FA, Leary GA, Baldwin WR, West DC, Box RA, Harris E, Johnson C. The transmission of refractive errors within Eskimo families. Am J Optom Arch Am Acad Optom. 46: 676-685, 1969.

Zadnik K, Mutti DO. How applicable are animal myopia models to human juvenile onset myopia. Vis Res. 1995; 35: 1283-8.

Zadnik K, Mutti DO. Refractive error changes in law students. Am J Optom Physiol Opt. 1987; 64: 558-61.

Zylbermann R, Landau D, Berson D. The influence of study habits on myopia in Jewish teenagers. J Pediatr Ophthalmol Strab. 1993; 30: 319-22.

CHAPTER 4
NEARWORK-INDUCED TRANSIENT MYOPIA

OVERVIEW

Studies on the dynamics of accommodation demonstrate that the system typically responds after a latency of 400 ms, exhibits a time constant of 200-250 ms, and reaches its final steady-state level in 4 or 5 time constants to a step input of blur (Campbell and Westheimer 1960, Ciuffreda and Kenyon 1983, see Ciuffreda 1991, in press, for detailed reviews). Thus, the total motor response (i.e., latency plus lens movement time) is completed in just over one second (Footnote 1). See Chapter 1.

However, most studies have shown that immediately following an extended and continuous near vision task, the final phase (i.e., the last 0.33D or so) of the actual accommodative movement time in response to a far target is prolonged (Footnote 2). This is reflected as a transient myopic shift in the measured post-task far point refraction. This short-term, nearwork-related, pseudomyopic far point shift has become known as "nearwork-induced transient myopia" (NITM) (Lancaster and Williams 1914, Ostberg 1980, Haider et al. 1980, Jaschinski-Kruza 1984, Ehrlich 1987, Fisher et al. 1987, Owens and Wolf-Kelly 1987, Gobba et al. 1988, Tan and O'Leary 1988, Rosenfield et al. 1992a and b, Blustein et al. 1993, Miwa and Tokoro 1993, Rosenfield and Ciuffreda 1994, Ong et al. 1994, Ciuffreda and Ordoñez 1995, Ciuffreda et al. 1996, Ong 1996, Ong et al. 1995, 1996). It may be operationally defined as the difference between the pre- and post-task distance refraction, with the pre-task level representing baseline refraction and the post-task level representing the refraction immediately following the near task. Because it may be influenced by external factors, this myopic shift is presumed to be environmental in nature, although a hereditary predisposition cannot be entirely ruled out. Lancaster and Williams (1914) suggested that it was probably lenticular in origin and due to an inability to relax accommodation rapidly and fully to the original baseline far point (i.e., an accommodative aftereffect or hysteresis phenomenon). It has an innervational and/or neuropharmacological origin.

NITM has been reported under both natural and experimental conditions following near vision tasks of various durations. It has been observed for near fixation durations as brief as 2-4 minutes (Ciuffreda et al. 1996) and as long as a full work day (Ostberg 1980). Its mean magnitude is approximately 0.33D, with a range from 0.12 to 1.30D. Its decay is characterized by an exponential function having a total time course ranging from 30 seconds for relatively short task durations (Rosenfield et al. 1992a) to as much as a few hours for longer near task durations (Ehrlich 1987).

The following is a critical review of this important basic and clinical area. We will first describe studies demonstrating NITM using either changes in visual acuity, contrast sensitivity function, or far point refraction to quantify this parameter, including its decay. Then studies not demonstrating NITM will be considered. Lastly, NITM will be discussed in more general terms in relation to tonic accommodation, accommodative hysteresis, accommodative disorders, and the possible role these factors may play in the development of clinical myopia. Pertinent details of the various studies are provided in Tables 4-1 and 4-2.

STUDIES DEMONSTRATING NITM (Table 4-1)

Visual Acuity as an Index of NITM

The literature documents numerous subjective accounts of blurred distance vision following near work which suggest a transient change in the far point (Ball 1982, Hung et al. 1986, Gilmartin and Bullimore 1987). In a study by Haider et al. (1980), changes in visual acuity were monitored and used to demonstrate this phenomenon. They investigated 22 subjects aged 21-45 years, consisting of 13 experimental subjects and 9 controls. The experimental group performed VDT (video display terminal) tasks for three continuous hours, while the control group performed varied office-related tasks over the same period which primarily involved different forms of typing. At the conclusion of the work period, NITM was inferred from subjective reports of a significant reduction in distance visual acuity in the experimental group, with recovery occurring within 10-15 minutes (Figure 4-1). No post-task reduction in visual acuity was found for the control group. Presumably the transient decrement of visual acuity in the experimental group was caused by the slight retinal defocus related to an inability to reduce accommodation rapidly back to the pre-task distance refractive level, and thus the blur-induced accommodative adaptation (i.e., an accommodative aftereffect or hysteresis) was evident. The authors estimated the myopic shift to be 0.25D, although further analyses derived from a comparison with their other related studies provided evidence of a somewhat greater magnitude. A study by Murch (1983) also showed a 15% reduction in visual acuity after the subjects performed work at a raster-scan display device. In addition, a comparative study was performed by Haider et al. (1980) to determine the effect of near task duration, as well as the use of continuous versus discontinuous periods of near work, on distance acuity. Smaller reductions

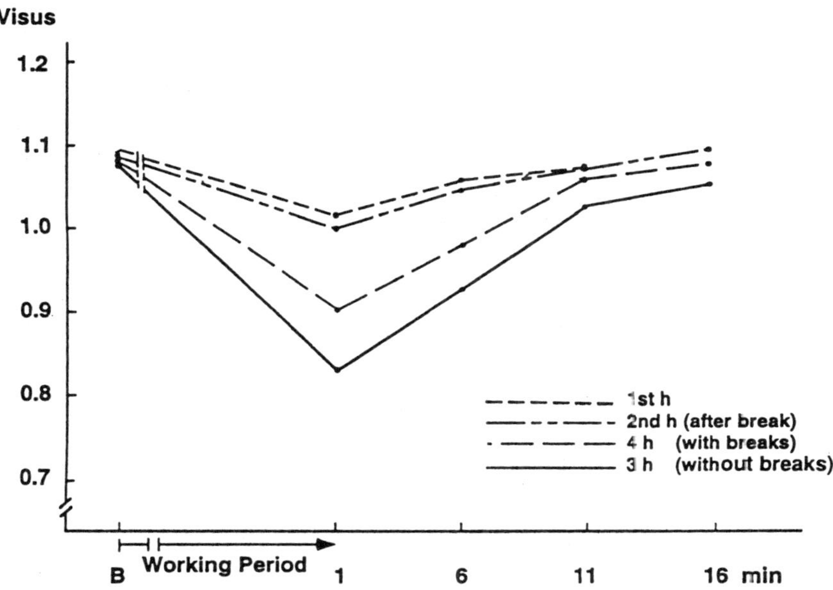

Figure 4-1 : Temporary myopization, expressed as mean value of visual acuity before and after working periods of different length, with and without rest periods (Reprinted with permission, Haider et al. 1980).

in visual acuity were demonstrated for the briefer work periods, as well as for those work periods interspersed with short rest periods. This is consistent with the advice optometrists provide their patients, especially college students and VDT users, who frequently complain of nearwork-related asthenopia.

Although a nearwork-induced far point change may generally translate into blurred distance vision if the depth-of-focus is exceeded, assessing visual acuity as an indicator of refractive change is clearly indirect. Furthermore, since such data are subjective in nature, there is an ever present risk of the various subjects adopting different criteria for detecting and reporting the presence of blur, as well as intersubject variability with respect to blur interpretation ability. This becomes even more critical if one considers the fact that this myopia is generally very small in magnitude and transient in nature. Moreover, the line gradations in standard visual acuity charts may not be as small as needed, and thus this may result in failure to detect more subtle refractive changes. In addition, since the perception of blur is constrained by the limits of the depth-of-focus, any small but consistent refractive change which still allows the retinal image of the object to fall within the depth-of-focus will not be evident to the individual.

TABLE 4-1: SUMMARY OF STUDIES DEMONSTRATING NEARWORK-INDUCED TRANSIENT MYOPIA

INVESTIGATOR (Year)	N/AGE (Yrs.)	APPARATUS	NEAR TASK PARADIGM	TARGET/ INSTRUCTIONS	TRANSIENT MYOPIA (D)	DECAY
Lancaster & Williams (1914)	NA/children to 60y	subjective measurement	at nearpoint for 45 min	small object/maintain clarity	1.30D	<15 min
Ostberg (1980)	29/18-50y	laser optometer	binocular at normal working distance for: ATC- 2 hrs TELE-8 hrs	VDT/under natural working conditions	ATC: 0.25D TELE: N.S.	>20 min
Haider, Kundi & Weibenbock (1980)	22/21-45y	visual acuity chart	binocular for 3 hrs	VDT/reading & copying	>0.25D	subjective recovery of distant vision in 10-15min
Jaschinski-Kruza (1984)	7/22-41y	contrast sensitivity measurement	binocular at normal working distance for 3 hrs	VDT/copying text	$\leq$ 0.50D	<15 min
Ehrlich (1987)	15/18-30y	Dioptron II infrared optometer	binocular at 20 cm (5D) for 2 hrs	number table (6/9) /visual search	0.29D	>1 hr
Fisher, Ciuffreda & Levine (1987)	48/21-35y	Hartinger coincidence optometer	monocular at nearpoint for 10 min	reduced Snellen/ maintain clarity	0.20D	N.A.
Owens & Kelly (1987)	28/17-22y	polarized vernier optometer	binocular at 20 cm (5D) for 1hr	text on hardcopy or VDT/reading	0.43D	>20 min
Gobba, Broglia, Sarti, Luberto & Cavallieri (1988)	38/19-52y	Canon R-1 infrared optometer	binocular at normal working distance for a full workday	VDT/data-acquisition tasks under natural working conditions	>0.50D	N.A.

Tan & O'Leary (1988)	18/19-27y	Polarized Scheiner Badal optometer	monocular at 25 cm (4D) for 15 min	text/reading	0.25D	N.A.
Rosenfield, Ciuffreda & Novogrodsky (1992a)	20/23-32y	Canon R-1 infrared optometer	binocular at 20 cm (5D) for 20 min	text/shading in letters	0.12D	complete after 30 sec
Rosenfield, Ciuffreda, Novogrodsky, Yu & Gillard (1992b) Duration:	10/NA	Canon R-1 infrared optometer	@ 25cm (4D) for 40 min (continuous or interrupted)	N.A.	0.20D	interrupted task: decay complete within 5 min
Accommodative Demand:	10/NA	Canon R-1 infrared optometer	monocular at 25 cm (4D), with +2D & +4D adds	N.A.	0.15D w/ 0.5mm pinhole, distance correction & +2D add N.S. w/ +4D add	N.A.
Miwa & Tokoro (1993)	19/19-20y	Nidek infrared autorefractometer	binocular at 30 cm w/-3D (6D) for 15 min	magazine/reading	0.21D	N.A.
Blustein, Rosenfield & Ciuffreda (1993)	15/N.A.	Canon R-1 infrared optometer	at 20 cm (5D) for 10 min	N.A.	0.30D	N.A.
Ong, Ciuffreda & Rosenfield (1994, 1996) Ong (1996)	16/21-33y	Canon R-1 infrared optometer	monocular & binocular at 6m & 40 cm (0 & 2.50D) w/ lenses & prisms for 10 min	matrix of numbers/adding	0.21 D	time constant of 51 sec
Rosenfield & Ciuffreda (1994)	12/21-25y	Canon R-1 infrared optometer	monocular at 20 cm (5D) for 10 min	matrix of numbers (N6)/reading or adding	0.23D	<40 sec with a time constant of 17 sec

Ciuffreda & Ordoñez (1995)	3/21-25y	Canon R-1 infrared optometer	binocular at 20 cm (5D) for 10 min	matrix of numbers/adding	0.93D	> 5 min
Ong, Ciuffreda & Rosenfield (1995)	15/22-39y	Canon R-1 infrared optometer	monocular at 20 cm (5D) for 10 min	matrix of numbers (6/9)/adding numbers	0.36D	time constant of 93 sec
Ciuffreda, Colburn & Wallis (1996)	12/21-28y	Canon R-1 infrared optometer	a) binocular at 20 cm (5D) for 0.25, 0.5, 1, 2, 4 & 8 min b) binocular at 6m, 33 & 20 cm (0, 3 & 5D) for 10 min	matrix of numbers/adding	0.30-0.60D	≤40 sec

---

N.A.= not available
N.S.= not significant

Contrast Sensitivity as an Index of NITM

In light of the small magnitude of this transient myopia, Jaschinski-Kruza (1984) regarded the use of conventional high contrast visual acuity tests as inadequate, as mentioned earlier. He therefore used contrast sensitivity to characterize subtle changes in spatial vision related to refractive state. Contrast thresholds were obtained from seven subjects engaged in computer-related, text-copying tasks for three continuous hours. This was measured by varying the contrast to a 10 cycle per degree (cpd), sinusoidally-modulated, vertically-oriented grating pattern viewed on a screen positioned 5 meters away. A comparison was made for thresholds obtained before and immediately after the near task. These pre-post measurements were also compared with thresholds that were determined with an additional -0.75D sphere in front of the subject's eye (i.e., their so-called compensated threshold), with the rationale being that any induced myopia could be compensated for by the introduction of the negative spherical lens, and any overcompensation by the spherical lens could be corrected by an appropriate amount of accommodative change. Therefore, any threshold difference obtained with and without the correcting lens would reflect the presence of some degree of induced myopia. The author reported a significant reduction of contrast sensitivity in 50% of the subjects following near work. Post-task uncompensated thresholds were almost twice that of the pre-task values, which corresponded to approximately a 0.50D myopic difference. Pre- and post-task compensated thresholds remained constant, therefore attesting to the fact that myopia was induced in an amount that was correctable by the -0.75 D spherical lens. Additional confirmation was provided by the presence of a difference between the post-task compensated and uncompensated thresholds. The post-task uncompensated threshold recovered to the pre-task level within 15 minutes. However, the use of contrast sensitivity rather than Snellen visual acuity as an index of NITM makes it difficult to translate this important finding into standard clinical terms.

Far Point Change as an Index of NITM

The optimal and most common method of measuring NITM is clearly by directly assessing any change in the distance refraction itself (i.e., far point of accommodation). The earliest observation of this phenomenon was documented in the now classic study by Lancaster and Williams (1914). The subject population ranged from a few young children of unspecified age up to adults 60 years of age. The far point was measured both prior to and at the end of a near task, with it being determined subjectively at both the far and near distances. At the far distance (6 m), it was specified as the maximum plus or minimum minus lens capable of producing maximum visual acuity. At the near distance, a suitable plus lens of known dioptric

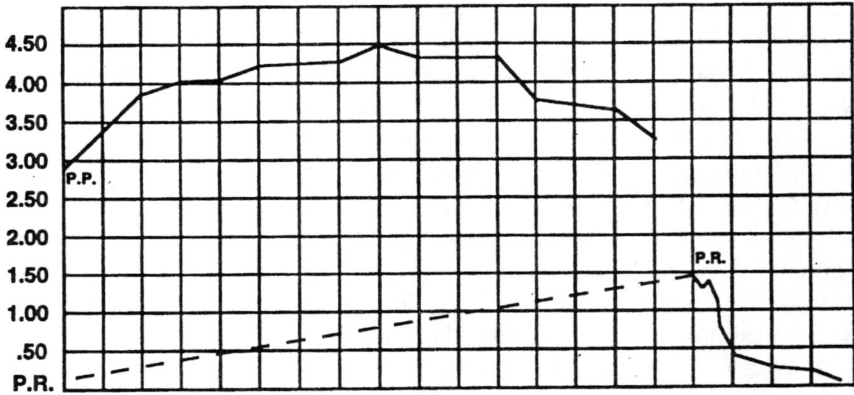

Figure 4-2 : Curve of punctum proximum, with continuous fixation of test object as near as possible for forty-five minutes, followed immediately by the curve of punctum remotum, with continuous fixation of the test object as far as possible, with a +2.00 D Badal lens system. Note the characteristic increase in power to accommodate, followed in this case by a definite falling off after about half an hour due to fatigue. The broken line shows how the punctum remotum becomes nearer during the very strong accommodation, suggesting contracture or spasm. It is followed by the curve showing recovery during the following fifteen minutes, with the punctum remotum gradually returning to normal. Observations made every 10 minutes, but this chart plotted from observations every 3 minutes, intermediate observations omitted. Each vertical space equals 0.50D, each horizontal space equals 3 minutes (Reprinted with permission, Lancaster and Williams 1914).

power was placed over the distance correction. The subject then determined the farthest optical distance that the test target could be clearly seen within this Badal optical system. The inducing task consisted of sustained focus on a small object positioned at the subject's near point for 45 minutes. Following this task, far point changes as large as 1.30D were observed, with a decay to pre-task baseline within 15 minutes (Figure 4-2). The authors attributed these temporary far point shifts to a strong contracture or spasm of accommodation which they referred to as "retarded relaxation," i.e., an inability to relax accommodation at far in the normal rapid manner as described earlier (i.e., 1 second or so). This is similar to what some symptomatic patients report following relatively brief periods of nearwork. This will also be elicited from such patients if high levels of accommodation are demanded of them during routine clinical testing, such as repeated near point of accommodation.

Little was done in this area using this parameter for almost the next seven decades, until computer display terminals became commonplace, and symptoms related to their use became prevalent. One of the first studies was that of Ostberg (1980), who investigated NITM in VDT users. The subjects were divided into 2 groups according to their visual task demand. The first group (n=9) consisted of air traffic controllers whose work involved continuous viewing of radar screens. The second group (n=20) consisted of traditional office workers and telephone directory service operators whose work involved less visually-taxing VDT-related tasks, with the latter perhaps being somewhat less continuous in nature. Working in their normal environment, steady-state accommodation for a distant target (6m) was measured statically and subjectively with a laser optometer. This represented the far point refraction. It was assessed both prior to and after two hours of near work in the first group of subjects, and prior to and at the end of the work day in the second group. The air traffic controllers exhibited a small but significant myopic far point shift of approximately 0.25D. The second group did not exhibit a significant shift. In addition, the post-task accommodative stimulus/response slope was significantly reduced in the first group, while it remained unchanged in the second group. The far point shift and the slope decrease both produced a transient increase in mean accommodative error. Ostberg attributed the differences between groups to the increased visual demand in the former group. It was commendable that this was a field study drawing from conditions present in the normal work environment rather than a laboratory environment. However, by the same token, this made comparison between the two groups of subjects more difficult. For example, proper control of test conditions, e.g., standardization of task, stimulus type, workload, etc., was not possible. Moreover, refraction was not measured at equal intervals in the two groups of subjects.

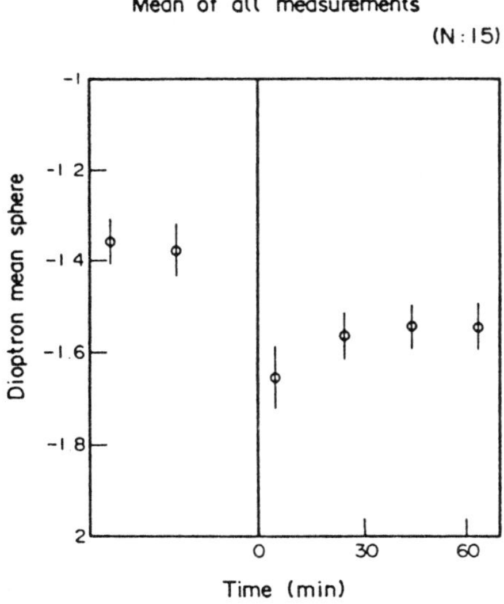

Figure 4-3 : Autorefractor measurement session means for 15 young, normal subjects who performed the two hour near task (20 cm). Error bars show ± 1 SEM for a typical subject's session. The vertical line represents the two hour near visual task. Data points to the left of the line show pre-task measurements (sessions 1 and 2). Data points to the right show post-task measurements (sessions 3-6). The near task induced an initial 0.29 diopter myopic change (Reprinted with permission, Ehrlich 1987).

An improvement over the methods used in the two previous studies was a direct and objective means of measuring the refractive state as conducted by Ehrlich (1987). He was the first to record NITM objectively, incorporating a Dioptron II infrared autorefractor under laboratory-controlled conditions. Fifteen young adult subjects performed a strenuous and continuous 2-

hour binocular near task at 20 cm (5D) involving a simple visual search paradigm consisting of counting the frequency of occurrence of a particular number within random number tables. Significant initial post-task myopic shifts with a mean of 0.29D were found (Figure 4-3). Ehrlich concluded that this induced transient myopia could be accounted for by an inward shift in tonic accommodation, with this amount being related to the initial pre-task tonic level: the higher the initial tonus level, the greater the change. He reasoned that with the continuous high level of accommodative effort necessary to maintain accurate focus, the accommodative hysteresis that was reflected in the (presumed) increased level of tonic accommodation developed as a consequence of increased innervation due to gradual fatiguing of the accommodative system. This myopic increase would then be carried over to distant viewing. With the tonic accommodative level shifting inward, presumably more "effort" would now be required to see a target clearly at distance, assuming this tonic level becomes the new "reference" point from which accommodative drive and effort are based. Thus, subjects exhibiting higher pre-task tonic levels would be predicted to demonstrate a greater amount of transient myopia (But see later discussion).

Another study also attributed changes in tonic accommodation per se to nearwork-related changes in this closed-loop accommodative response at far. Owens and Wolf-Kelly (1987) found a myopic shift over a range of accommodative stimulus levels (0 to 4D) following an extended near visual task (Figure 4-4). Using a static polarized vernier optometer, their measurements included the monocular far point, the monocular accommodative stimulus/response function, and tonic accommodation both prior to and after a binocular near task. Subjects were required to read text on either a VDT

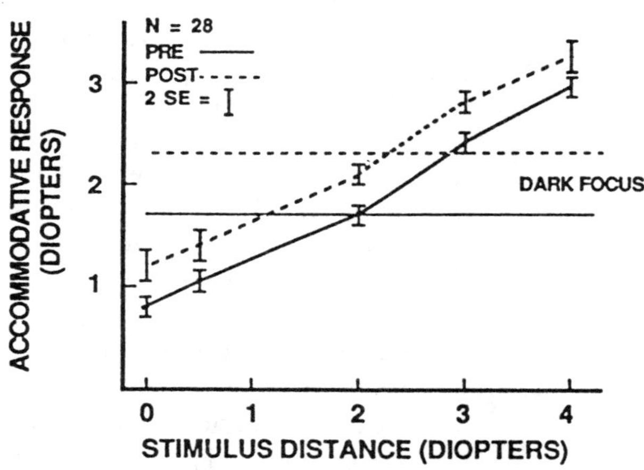

Figure 4-4 : Mean dark focus and accommodative response functions before (solid lines) and after (dashed lines) subjects read for 1 hr at a distance of 20 cms. Both the dark focus and accommodative responses showed significant shifts in the myopic direction. Vertical bars indicate two SEM's. Linear regressions showed that the mean accommodative response functions before and after reading were: $f(x) = 0.54x + 0.76$ ($r^2 = 0.992$) and $f(x) = 0.52x + 1.16$ ($r^2 = 0.994$), respectively (Reprinted with permission, Owens and Wolf-Kelly 1987).

screen or as hardcopy at a distance of 20 cm (5D) for one continuous hour. A substantial closed-loop mean transient myopic shift at far averaging 0.43D was found following the task, with this being the greatest group mean myopic shift reported in any study using visually-normal individuals. Furthermore, the entire accommodative stimulus/response function was biased upward by approximately 0.30D, again reflecting the phenomenon of transient myopia and representing increased accommodative error, but now at all stimulus levels.

A study by Fisher et al. (1987) found similar results using a slightly different paradigm. Subjects were required to maintain a 20/20 row of Snellen letters in focus at all times. The Snellen target was presented monocularly for 10 minutes at the subject's near point. The far point was measured subjectively with a static Hartinger coincidence optometer. Following near fixation, a significant group mean myopic shift of 0.20 D was observed. The data were then divided into four subgroups consisting of 12 subjects each based on their refractive error. These included emmetropes (± 0.75D), hyperopes (>+0.75D), and high (>-4D) and low (>-0.75D but ≤ -4D) myopes. However, now there was no significant transient myopic shift observed for any subgroup. This may be accounted for by the relatively small sample size of each subgroup, thereby reducing statistical power. In addition, this was compounded by the relatively small magnitude of the transient myopia, and thus there was less likelihood for any differential subgroup effect to be evident.

Myopic shifts were also reported in an investigation by Gobba et al. (1988) on 38 VDT data-acquisition operators. Distance refraction was assessed objectively with a Canon R-1 infrared autorefractor both prior to and at the conclusion of the workshift, the latter of which varied between two and seven hours. Significant far point changes greater than 0.50D were observed in 25% of the subjects. However, some subjects used their habitual prescription/viewing condition. Consequently, a few unspecified subjects may have been left with an uncorrected (in part or total) refractive error at either distance or near that could contaminate the results. Furthermore, the criterion for significance established by the authors was arbitrary and relatively large, i.e., only a difference of at least 0.50D was considered "significant," and thus standard statistical testing was not employed. Since information regarding response variability was not available, it is not known if such a criterion was appropriate. In addition, since NITM is presumably lenticular in origin, using a subject population which included presbyopes (ages ranged from 19-52 years) having considerably reduced or even absence of accommodative ability would tend to reduce the mean myopic aftereffect.

Tan and O'Leary (1988) compared the far point refraction following two conditions. Eighteen subjects were required to view a commercial television

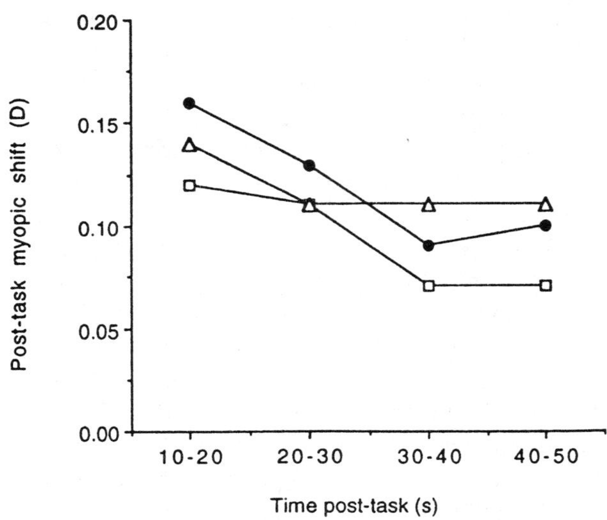

Figure 4-5 : Mean post-task myopic shift during the 10 to 50s immediately after completion of a 20 min near-vision task (viewing distance = 20 cm) for the three prism (disparity-vergence) conditions: ●, base-out; ❑, zero; Δ, base-in. There was no significant difference between the results for the three vergence stimuli. However, the myopic shift observed during the 10 to 20s post-task period was statistically significant, while the shifts for the 30 to 50s post-task interval were not significant. Error bars have been omitted for clarity, but SEMs were of the order of ± 0.06 D for all conditions (Reprinted with permission, Rosenfield et al. 1992a).

broadcast at 6 m, as well as to read a book positioned at 25 cm (4D), for a continuous period of 15 minutes. A polarized Scheiner-Badal subjective optometer was used to measure the far point statically. A mean myopic shift of 0.25D was reported upon completion of the near task. In contrast, no significant change in far point was found following the distance task. They too, like both Ehrlich (1987) and Owens and Wolf-Kelly (1987), attributed this refractive shift to an actual change in tonic accommodation.

Similarly, Rosenfield et al. (1992a) used a Canon R-1 infrared autorefractor and found a myopic shift following a 20-minute binocular near task. The experiment was comprised of three conditions. With the accommodative demand maintained at 5D, the vergence stimulus was either 5 meter angles (congruent condition) or varied with the introduction of base-out or base-in ophthalmic prisms (non-congruent condition) to drive vergence accommodation (Kran and Ciuffreda 1988), the prism magnitude of which was one-third of the subject's directional vergence range. Subjects were required to perform a fine hand-eye coordination task, i.e., to shade in specific letters embedded in a matrix of near-threshold letters. Statistically equivalent myopic shifts were observed for all three conditions over the entire post-task period, with a small but significant group mean initial post-task shift of 0.12D (Figure 4-5). Clearly, changes in vergence accommodative drive under closed-loop viewing conditions had little differential effect on NITM. The induced myopic shift dissipated reasonably rapidly, with baseline being attained statistically within the initial 30-50 second post-task interval.

In a separate study, Rosenfield et al. (1992b) attempted to determine the differential effect of blur-driven accommodation on NITM. Ten subjects performed a monocular near task at a distance of 25 cm under four conditions, namely : (1) through their distance correction to obtain the full blur stimulus, (2) through a 0.5mm pinhole to negate the full blur stimulus, (3) through an add of +2D to reduce the blur stimulus by 50%, and (4) through an add of +4D to reduce the blur stimulus by 100%. Once again, a Canon R-1 static infrared optometer was used to record the far point changes objectively. Significant initial group mean myopic shifts of approximately 0.15D were observed for all conditions except for the last one, as the +4D add effectively canceled any blur stimulus/drive to accommodation. These results suggest that the *full* blur stimulus must be negated to prevent the occurrence of transient myopia. Interestingly, in the pinhole condition, no blur was present, but NITM still occurred due to the proximal accommodative drive that was allowed to become manifested under the open-loop accommodative viewing condition (Rosenfield and Gilmartin 1990, Rosenfield et al. 1991, Hung et al. 1996). Furthermore, the authors concluded that the transient myopia was related to the aggregate (i.e., blur plus proximity) within-task accommodative response. In this same report, they also investigated NITM as a function of task duration. A near task (25 cm) was performed for 40 minutes, either continuously or in four 10-minute sessions separated by 5-minute rest periods. Statistically equivalent and significant initial group mean myopic far point shifts of approximately 0.20D were found. Periodic interruption of the task had no effect on NITM. However, in the latter condition, the 5-minute rest periods were sufficient to enable the transient myopia to decay fully, whereas such full decay was not found for the continuous task. This was similar to that found by Haider et al. (1980) as described earlier using contrast sensitivity as the test probe. And, this is similar to what optometrists have been advising patients to do to reduce their nearwork-related asthenopia; but here there is now objective evidence showing that frequent rest periods also allow NITM to dissipate fully and prevent the occurrence of any pseudomyopia (Ong and Ciuffreda 1995) and perhaps even permanent myopia (Mei and Rong 1994).

Miwa and Tokoro (1993) obtained far point myopic shifts that were of a similar magnitude to the earlier studies. They had 19 young-adult subjects perform a binocular reading task for 15 minutes. The reading material was positioned 30 cm away, and -3D spherical lenses were worn over the subject's habitual distance correction. This effectively created an accommodative stimulus of approximately 6D, thus making the test condition markedly non-congruent. The post-task far point exhibited a significant mean myopic shift of 0.21D. When the subjects were further divided into two groups based on the magnitude of their habitual myopia (either greater or less than 2D), a similar amount of myopic shift was found for each group. Thus, the magnitude of their permanent myopia did not have any effect on NITM.

To determine the effect of cognitive demand on NITM, the latter was recently assessed following a 10-minute monocular task performed at 20 cm (Rosenfield and Ciuffreda 1994). A Canon R-1 infrared autorefractor was once again used to measure far point changes objectively. The target consisted of a matrix of near threshold sized numbers. The cognitive demand was systematically varied between three levels: (1) low cognitive demand: subjects were instructed simply to read the numbers aloud, (2) moderate cognitive demand: subjects were instructed to add pairs of single digit numbers, and (3) high cognitive demand: subjects were instructed to add a series of four paired numbers. A significant initial group mean transient myopic shift of 0.25D was induced in all conditions, with the subsequent decay to pre-task refractive baseline being completed within 40 seconds. No difference in magnitude was found between conditions, thereby suggesting that cognitive demand level was not instrumental in inducing differential NITM under normal closed-loop viewing conditions. Again, the notion of the aggregate accommodative response was invoked. And, it should be recalled that in normals the depth-of-focus limits any substantial changes in magnitude of steady-state accommodation from occurring. Thus, perhaps an open-loop near accommodative paradigm should be used to elicit the full potential impact of cognitive demand on this parameter.

More recently, Ong et al. (1995) assessed NITM objectively with a Canon R-1 infrared optometer to determine the role of target proximity on NITM. Equidioptric targets of 5 D were monocularly viewed at either a far distance of 6 m through a -5D lens over the distance refractive correction (blur only condition) or a near distance of 20 cm (blur plus proximal condition) (Rosenfield et al. 1991). Young adult subjects (n=15) were required to add a series of near threshold-sized numbers to ensure attention and accuracy of focus for the test duration of 10 minutes. A significant initial group mean myopic shift of approximately 0.3 D was observed for each condition. Since the magnitude of NITM was similar for both conditions, NITM thus again appeared to be related to the overall (or aggregate) drive of the accommodative system independent of the type of input stimulus (Rosenfield et al. 1992b, Rosenfield and Ciuffreda 1994).

Only one study has been done on individuals with symptoms of blur at distance following a short period of near work. Using an NITM near task paradigm and Canon device similar to that described earlier in normals, Ciuffreda and Ordoñez (1995) tested 3 symptomatic subjects. In contrast to

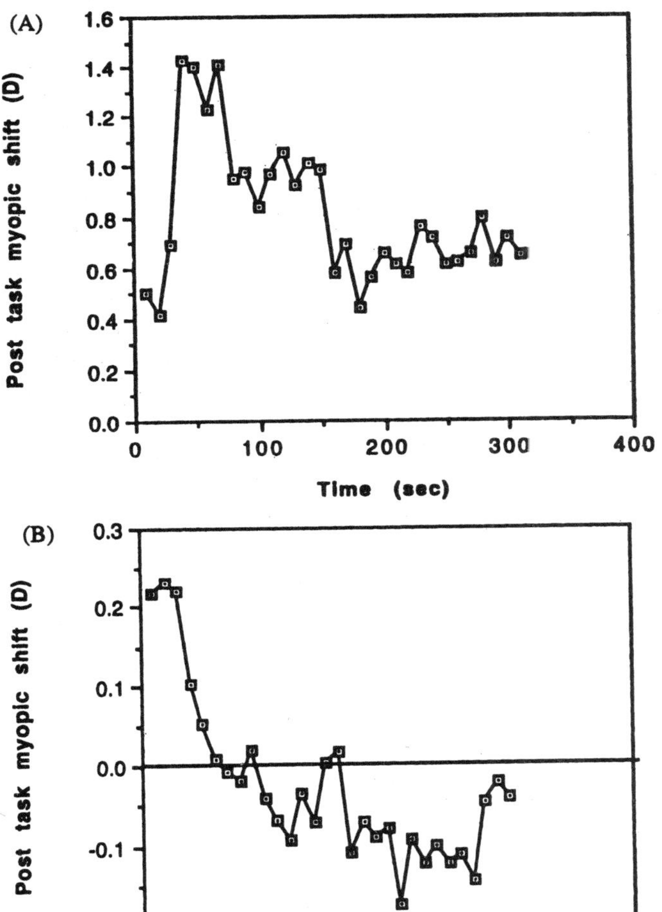

Figure 4-6 : NITM as a function of time. (A) In a subject with the symptom of transient blur at distance following a short period of near work; the large initial NITM response does not reduce to the pre-task refractive state (zero baseline) during the subsequent 5-minute post-task period, and (B) In an asymptomatic subject; the 0.25D initial NITM decays to baseline in approximately 30 sec, with most subsequent data points falling within the ± 0.1D pre-task refractive state "noise level" (i.e. ± 1 SD) (Reprinted with permission, Ciuffreda and Ordoñez 1995).

asymptomatic individuals who showed (1) small initial post-task myopic shift without noticing the perception of blur, (2) rapid dissipation or decay (<30 sec or so) of this initial effect, and (3) little response variability of the initial effect and exponential decay, the symptomatic subjects exhibited (1) large initial post-task myopic shift concurrent with the perception of transient blur, (2) slowed dissipation of this initial effect with little sensation of blur, and finally (3) increased response variability of the initial effect as well as the decay (Figure 4-6). These results are consistent with the subjects' symptoms, as well as the overall clinical picture. Experiments in progress (Ciuffreda and Ordoñez) have demonstrated that simple accommodative facility therapy can enhance the decay of NITM, as well as improve related clinical findings and markedly reduce symptoms.

Employing a similar NITM experimental protocol, Ong et al. (1994, 1996) and Ong (1996) investigated the relative contribution of blur, disparity, and proximity on NITM. With the use of spherical lenses and prisms, targets at a far distance of 6 m (0.16D) and a near distance of 40 cm (2.5D) were presented to create either congruent or non-congruent conditions of blur, disparity and proximal stimuli. The tasks were performed under either closed or open-loop conditions. To ensure maintenance of clarity of vision, the 16 late-onset myopes were instructed to perform mental addition of near threshold numbers for 10 minutes continuously, while their pre-and post-task far point of accommodation was assessed objectively with a Canon R-1 infrared optometer. The study demonstrated that a range of statistically significant transient myopia (0.18-0.39D) was induced for the various conditions. Furthermore, such statistically significant shifts were demonstrated only for those conditions that stimulated blur to a non-zero level. Conversely, no refractive shifts were evident when the blur-driven component was minimally stimulated regardless of the contribution of the disparity-vergence and proximal accommodative components. In addition, the stimulation of the latter two components to a level or direction different from that of the blur-driven component resulted in either an enhanced myopic or hyperopic shift, respectively. More specifically, greater myopic shifts were demonstrated for viewing paradigms in which the disparity

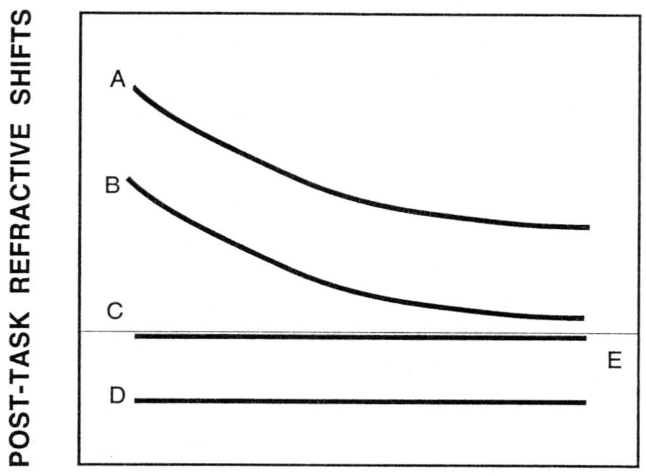

Figure 4-7 : A schematic representation of various post-task refractive response profiles differentiated by the input of blur-driven accommodation. The thin "E" line represents baseline refraction. Refractive shifts above and below the baseline are myopic and hyperopic in direction, respectively. Curve "A" depicts the condition of enhanced blur. Curve "B" represents the normal binocular congruent viewing condition whereby all components are equally stimulated to a non-zero level. Its analogous condition whereby all components are stimulated at zero levels is plotted as curve "C". Finally, curve "D" characterizes the condition of inhibition of the blur stimulus.

vergence and proximal components were non-congruently stimulated with respect to the blur-driven component by virtue of the additional defocus introduced by means of minus lenses. Conversely, hyperopic shifts were observed following viewing conditions in which plus lenses were introduced to create non-congruent demands with respect to the disparity vergence and proximal components. A summarized schematic representation of the various response categories differentiated by the magnitude and direction of the blur input is depicted in Figure 4-7. Hence, the results suggest that blur-driven accommodation was the primary determinant of NITM, and that the contribution of disparity and proximity was relatively small under normal closed-loop viewing conditions. This is consistent with the notion that blur is the stimulus to accommodation (Morgan 1968, Ciuffreda 1991, in press). These results were confirmed by model computations (See Appendix 1).

Lastly, recent experiments in our laboratory on nearwork-induced transient myopia have demonstrated the following: (1) after only 4 minutes of sustained binocular nearwork, significant NITM was found (Ciuffreda et al. 1996), (2) for extended 4 hour periods, 3 response subgroups were found: some showed no NITM, while others showed either normal NITM with subsequent decay or NITM that was maintained during the entire test period, (3) focusing on either a 3 or 5 D target resulted in similar amounts of NITM (Ciuffreda et al. 1996), and (4) *myopes were particularly susceptible to NITM*, whereas hyperopes and emmetropes were not (Ciuffreda and Wallis, in preparation).

Potential Problems with the Above Studies

In general, the NITM reported by the above studies in primarily visually-normal individuals was small in magnitude. This comes as no surprise. Since NITM can only be studied with accommodation in the closed-loop mode, i.e., with normal blur feedback, such aftereffects are of necessity somewhat restricted in magnitude due to limitations imposed by the depth-of-focus of the eye. If this were not true, subjects would report transient blur at far much more frequently.

Unfortunately, in almost all of the studies, the actual accommodative response during the near task was not assessed. Therefore, most of the findings were based on the assumption that accommodation was responding more or less accurately to the stimulus demand. This appears to be a reasonable assumption, however, since clarity of vision was subjectively monitored and maintained for the small detailed targets. Moreover, in a few studies (Ong 1996, Ciuffreda et al. 1996), the accommodative response during the inducing task was monitored objectively in several subjects, and it was found to be within normal limits.

Induction of small amounts of NITM under the diverse conditions of the various experiments suggests generality of the basic phenomenon. However, by combining results across all subjects, the effect might be reduced in both magnitude and duration. It may be more clearly manifested within subgroups who exhibit inherent differences in susceptibility to NITM, and this notion warrants further careful consideration and testing with various clinical populations; for example, those with near esophoria who are at risk of becoming myopic should prove to be an interesting population (Goss 1991). Clearly, averaging data across *all* subjects would reduce this already small and transient aftereffect.

Decay Characteristics of NITM

The decay of NITM to the pre-task baseline refraction exhibited an exponential function in visually-normal individuals. It appeared to be more strongly affected by task duration than either the initial magnitude of NITM or the task demand. Variable decay times were found despite similar accommodative demands and instrumentation. A majority of the studies used objective infrared autorefractors and a near task distance of 20 cm (5 D) with their young adult visually-normal populations. While task durations lasting from 10 to 20 minutes generally resulted in a rapid and precipitous return to baseline (typically in 30 seconds or so), tasks of extended durations (>40 minutes) generally resulted in more prolonged aftereffects (minutes). For example, Ehrlich (1987) found that following a 2-hour continuous near task, the post-task decay was still significantly above baseline after one hour (Figure 4-3). On the other hand, using a shorter task duration (20 minutes), Rosenfield et al. (1992a) reported that the myopic shifts had rapidly dissipated and were not significantly above baseline within the initial 30-50 second post-task interval (Figure 4-5). The presence of a relation between the time course of NITM decay and task duration supports the speculation that repeated occurrences of transient myopia may lead to more permanent forms of myopia, as mentioned earlier. The decay profile also appeared to be related to the nature of the accommodative stimulus. More specifically, its time course seemed to vary with the magnitude of target defocus. For stimuli consisting of a predominantly blur component, a protracted decay was observed. See later discussion.

In addition, the decay pattern also appeared to be related to symptomatology associated with near work. Results from a recent study provided evidence for a greater transient myopic shift (up to 1.50D), prolonged decay (>5 minutes), and increased response variability (ranging from no aftereffect to a large aftereffect) on different test sessions in a small sample of such symptomatic subjects using our basic near test paradigm and a Canon R-1 autorefractor (Ciuffreda and Ordoñez 1995, in progress) (Figure 4-6).

A complicating factor is the presence of blur visual feedback at distance. In the numerous studies on simple decay of accommodative adaptation (Rosenfield et al. 1994b), this measurement was taken in total darkness, and thus simply reflected the time constant of the slow accommodative adaptive loop (Hung 1992) (Figure 4-8). In contrast, for the decay of NITM, this profile reflected both this internal time constant as well as the presence of blur visual feedback and its interactive effect on the accommodative adaptive loop dynamics, resulting in the post-task refractive state at far (i.e., far point of accommodation) measured in the experiments. Whether a subject simply "relaxed" during the decay period and had reflexive far accommodation activated, or attempted to exert some voluntary control to clear the blur more rapidly, could alter this response profile dramatically. Thus, this important issue remains unresolved. Furthermore, its decay characteristics may also be related to the etiology of more long-term forms of myopia. See later discussion.

STUDIES NOT DEMONSTRATING NITM (Table 4-2)

However, not all studies have found induced transient myopia following near work irrespective of the parameter being measured. These will be discussed in detail in this section. See Table 4-2.

TABLE 4-2: SUMMARY OF STUDIES NOT DEMONSTRATING NEARWORK-INDUCED TRANSIENT MYOPIA

INVESTIGATOR (Year)	N/AGE (Yrs.)	APPARATUS	NEAR TASK/ PARADIGM	TARGET INSTRUCTIONS
Dainoff & Happ (1981)	23/N.A.	visual acuity test with a visual screening device	binocular at normal working distance for a day	VDT/ work environment
Nyman, Knave & Voss (1985)	505/20-60y	Dioptron II infrared optometer	binocular at normal working distance for 5 hrs	VDT/ work environment
Pigion & Miller (1985)	20/18-23y	laser optometer	monocular at 30cm for 1 hour	text on slides/read aloud
Ebenholtz & Zander (1987)	17/17-21y	laser optometer	at near point for 8 min	B/W horizontal gratings/sustained focus
Shen, Chiu, Wang & Ko (1988)	23/19-36y	visual acuity test	binocular at normal working distance for a day	VDT/ work environment
Gur & Ron (1992)	26/24-43y	contrast sensitivity test	binocular at normal working distance for a day	VDT/ work environment
Harrington, Watanabe, Jiang & White (1992)	16/N.A.	Canon R-1 infrared optometer	binocular at 17cm (6D) for 20 min	computer game/interactive playing

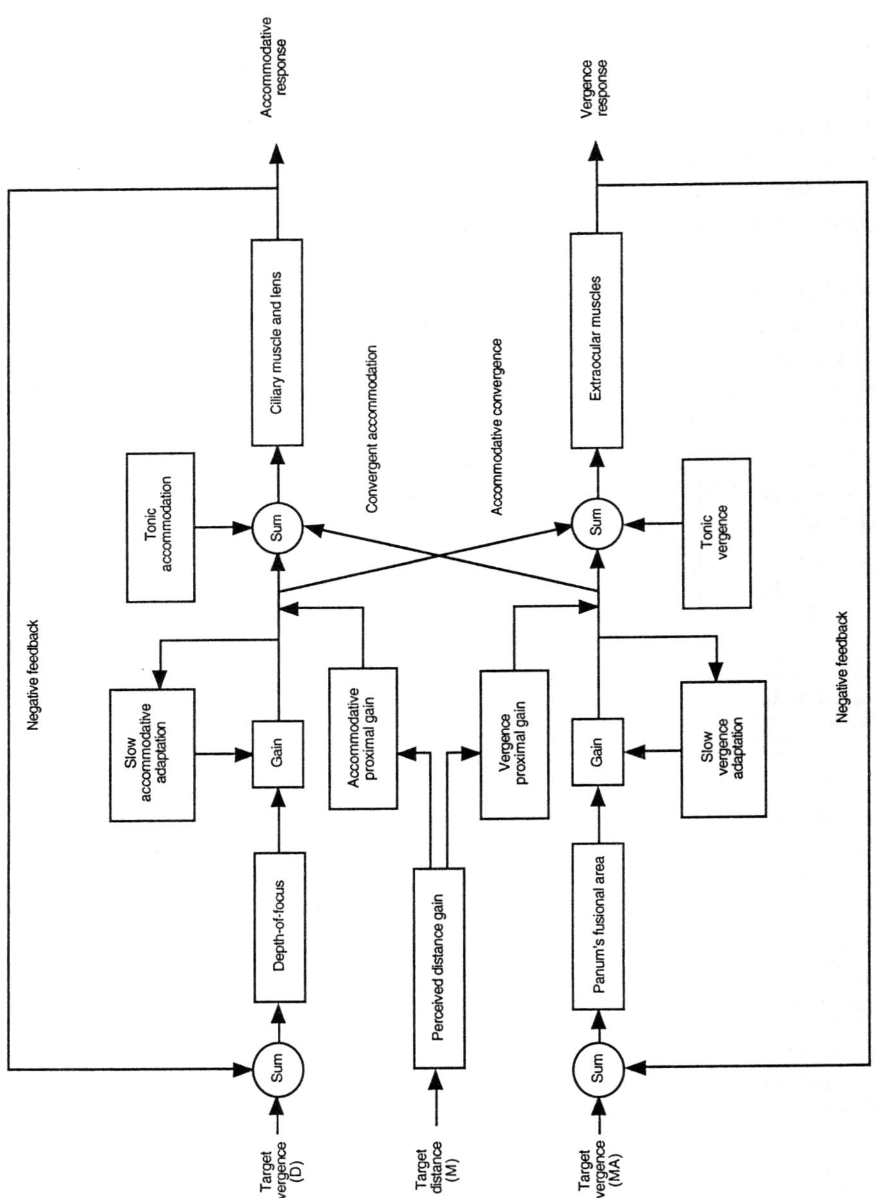

Figure 4-8: Comprehensive Hung-Ciuffreda-Rosenfield static model of accommodation and vergence showing blur, disparity and proximity inputs and related pathways. All inputs are positive except for the negative feedback. SUM= input summing junction (Reprinted with permission, Ong and Ciuffreda 1995).

Visual Acuity as an Index of NITM

In an investigation of nearwork-induced visual acuity changes, Dainoff and Happ (1981) studied 23 library employees whose main task consisted of data entry with 75% of their working time involving the use of VDTs. Visual acuity was assessed binocularly over a period of a week using an industrial screening device. Subjects were trained to take their own measurements prior to and after the first and second work shift each day. No changes in visual acuity were observed following the first work shift nor at the end of the day. According to the authors, the lack of any transient myopia was most probably due to the allowance of informal rest periods, and this is indeed a likely possibility as described earlier. For example, Haider (1980) showed that work periods interspersed with rest periods resulted in visual acuity changes of a lesser magnitude (Figure 4-1). Moreover, Rosenfield et al. (1992b) demonstrated that the interposition of a 5-min rest interval for every 10 minutes of nearwork time allowed a complete recovery of any transient myopic changes. Clearly, incorporation of brief but frequent rest intervals during the work day in individuals performing prolonged nearwork, such as VDT operators, would be of short and possibly even long-term benefit. Aside from this, other factors may have come into play as well. Screening devices are designed to detect relatively gross abnormalities. Since any induced changes in visual acuity following nearwork are generally subtle, the use of a screening device is not optimal. Moreover, allowing subjects to take their own measurements may have resulted in measurement inaccuracies, as well as changes in criteria for determining visual acuity.

The work by Shen et al. (1988) demonstrated similar results. Visual acuity was compared prior to and following a day of VDT work in 23 young adult students. They reported that no significant differences in visual acuity were found, although no actual data were presented. The authors indicated that no change in the usual daily work pattern was attempted. Therefore, rest periods were allowed as needed. Again, this may in part explain the absence of induced visual acuity changes.

Contrast Sensitivity as an Index of NITM

In a study of contrast sensitivity, Gur and Ron (1992) found no changes in this parameter at the end of the work day. The experimental population consisted of thirteen VDT operators who were involved in 5 to 6 hours of daily computer graphic tasks. They were compared to a group of control subjects consisting of office employees whose tasks only involved brief periods of reading, writing, and the use of VDTs. Monocular contrast sensitivity was evaluated with a Vision Contrast Test System Chart at 3 m. This was performed before and 15 to 20 minutes after the conclusion of the work day. No significant group differences were found, nor were any patterns of variation detected between the two groups of subjects. However, blurred distant vision after the work day was reported more frequently in VDT users than in the general office worker. Unfortunately, this was not quantified. The major factor responsible for the absence of NITM was probably due to the delay in obtaining post-task measurements. Since nearwork-induced changes in any such parameter are short-lived (i.e., generally less than a minute) (Rosenfield et al. 1992a, Rosenfield and Ciuffreda 1994, Ong et al. 1994), measuring contrast sensitivity 15 to 20 minutes after work completion probably allowed dissipation of any transient effects.

Far Point Change as an Index of NITM

The use of the far point of accommodation as a reference baseline for measuring NITM also yielded similar results. In an attempt to determine the impact of VDT's on various ocular functions, Nyman et al. (1985) assessed the refractive state of 505 subjects using a Dioptron autorefractometer. Measurements were obtained either immediately prior to or at commencement of work and immediately prior to the conclusion of the work day. A total of 379 VDT operators was examined, and their data were compared to that of 126 general office employees. No differences in distance refraction were found between the two specified occasions nor between the two groups of subjects.

Pigion and Miller (1985) examined 20 young adult emmetropes with a laser optometer. Different viewing conditions were presented to the subjects, but the one of particular relevance here involved a near task which consisted of a full hour of reading. The reading material was printed on slides and was positioned at 30 cm (3.3D). Subjects performed the task monocularly. No statistically significant difference in far point was evident following the task. According to the authors, the absence of a change in far point could have been due to the following two reasons: (1) the task demand or task duration was of an insufficient magnitude as to produce any changes. However, there is ample evidence that goes against this notion. Contrary to these findings, studies by Ong et al. (1994, 1996) and Ong (1996) demonstrated NITM despite the use of a task of lesser dioptric demand and duration. Several other studies which used tasks performed at normal working distances have also found myopic shifts (Ostberg 1980, Haider et al. 1980, Jaschinski-Kruza 1984, Gobba et al. 1988). Although the exact target distance in these studies (Ostberg 1980, Haider et al. 1980, Jaschinski-Kruza 1984, Gobba et al. 1988) was never specified, one may more or less presume that the dioptric demand is comparable to that of Pigion and Miller (1985). On the other hand, using tasks of much shorter duration also elicited transient changes in the far point (Lancaster and Williams 1914, Fisher et al. 1987, Tan and O'Leary 1988, Rosenfield et al. 1992a and b, Blustein et al. 1993, Miwa and Tokoro 1993, Rosenfield and Ciuffreda 1994, Ong et al. 1994, Ciuffreda and Ordoñez 1995, Ong et al. 1995, 1996, Ciuffreda et al. 1996, Ong 1996), although with a few exceptions (Ong et al. 1994, Ong 1996, Ong et al. 1996, Ong 1996, Ciuffreda et al. 1996), these studies involved tasks of greater dioptric demand. (2) these effects are better demonstrated under binocular viewing conditions, thus implicating vergence accommodation in addition to blur-driven accommodation. However, Ong et al. (1994, 1996) and Ong (1996) showed no difference in the magnitude of NITM under either binocular or monocular conditions. Moreover, despite the use of monocular tasks in several studies, NITM was nonetheless demonstrated (Fisher et al. 1987, Tan and O'Leary 1988, Rosenfield et al. 1992b, Rosenfield and Ciuffreda 1994, Ong et al. 1994, 1995, 1996, Ong 1996). Furthermore, recent work shows that the impact of vergence accommodation on NITM (Rosenfield et al. 1992a, Ong et al. 1994, 1996, Ong 1996) and on the overall accommodative response (Ong 1996) is minimal.

A study by Ebenholtz and Zander (1987) subjectively measured the far point with a laser optometer. Seventeen young adult emmetropes participated in the study. Focus at the near point of accommodation was sustained for a period of 8 minutes. No mean far point shift was demonstrated following the task. However, this might be related to either one of the following two factors. First, the post-task far point was always assessed *after* the post-task tonic accommodation measurements were taken, and thus the experimental design technique of counterbalancing was not applied. And, second, Ebenholtz and Zander (1987) used a laser optometer, which involved a comparatively long post-task measurement period. Thus, these two factors may have allowed dissipation of any induced myopia to occur prior to completion of the measurements.

More recently, Harrington et al. (1992) measured the accommodative stimulus/response function prior to and following a near vision task in a group of subjects comprised of emmetropes and late-onset myopes. The near vision task consisted of playing an interactive computer game at a distance equivalent to 6D for a duration of 20 minutes. The pre- and post-task accommodative stimulus/response functions were assessed objectively using a Canon R-1 infrared optometer. The accommodative stimulus consisted of a 20/100 computer-generated target which was physically positioned in space to encompass a stimulus range of 0.25 to 6D. No changes in accommodation were reported following the task. The absence of any post-task changes in accommodation could be due to the sequence of the measurements obtained. It appeared that the post-task accommodative stimulus/response function was always measured following that of post-task tonic accommodation. As discussed earlier, this would potentially allow sufficient time for dissipation of any accommodative aftereffects. In fact, the authors suggested that their finding might be due to the rapid decay of accommodative adaptation. And, related to this, there was no counterbalancing. See Chapter 2 for further discussion.

In summary, the inability to observe any consistent reductions in either visual acuity (Dainoff and Happ 1981, Shen et al. 1988), contrast sensitivity (Gur and Ron 1992), or myopic far point shifts (Nyman et al. 1985, Pigion and Miller 1985, Ebenholtz and Zander 1987, Harrington et al. 1992) could be attributed to a variety of methodological problems. These included lack of counterbalancing (Ebenholtz and Zander 1987; Harrington et al. 1992), delay in obtaining measurements (Ebenholtz and Zander 1987, Gur and Ron 1992, Harrington et al. 1992), use of non-optimal instrumentation (Dainoff and Happ 1981, Ebenholtz and Zander 1987), and the introduction of rest intervals (Dainoff and Happ 1981, Shen et al. 1988). However, some of the studies that demonstrated NITM could also be criticized for having one or more of the above methodological problems. Given the subtle and transient nature of NITM, the presence of such problems probably reduced the likelihood of detecting NITM. This could account for some of the inconsistency in results, even in two studies using similar (and perhaps even flawed) methodologies. In addition, since NITM is relatively small in magnitude, its decay time course relatively brief, and its occurrence possibly related to a differential susceptibility across individuals, it comes as no surprise that not all studies exhibited this phenomenon. Nor is it surprising that it may in fact not be present at all times for all individuals under all conditions. Furthermore, subgroup analysis may have been a more appropriate way to handle the data in some of the studies, including those with both positive and negative results, as averaging across subjects who showed no myopic shift along with those showing the typical small shift would reduce the overall group effect.

TONIC ACCOMMODATION, ACCOMMODATIVE ADAPTATION, NEARWORK-INDUCED TRANSIENT MYOPIA AND PERMANENT AXIAL-BASED MYOPIA

Tonic Accommodation and Axial Length

Historically, researchers focused on tonic accommodation as a potential factor in the development of myopia. This was based on van Alphen's ideas (1961, also see Holm 1926 in Chapter 5). He proposed an ocular-based physiological negative feedback mechanism for the process of emmetropization. He speculated that there were various "factors" involved. Factor S or the "size" factor determined the inherent overall size of the eye independent of its refraction. It was responsible for the relation between corneal power and axial length. Hence, larger eyes tended to be associated with flatter corneas. Factor P or the "stretch" factor determined the relation between axial length, lens power, and anterior chamber depth. Thus, there was a trend for larger eyes to have flatter lenses as well as increased anterior chamber depths. In effect, the final eye size was believed to be the result of the interaction between the size (S) and the stretch (P) factors. While the basic size was genetically-determined, stretch depended on the intraocular pressure and the elasticity of the ocular coats. Eyes of any sizes would have to stretch to achieve emmetropization. The stretching that resulted in ametropia was accounted for by factor R. Thus, R represented the degree of adjustment of P relative to S, and thus was the determinant of the final refraction. In this regard, the degree as well as the mechanism of stretch becomes crucial in the development of axial myopia.

Van Alphen introduced the concept that this scleral stretch was determined by the tonus of the ciliary muscle-choroid complex. According to his theory, the choroid and the ciliary muscle were regarded as a single physiological unit. The overall "tone" of the ciliary muscle-choroid envelope was determined by the physiological innervational tonus of the ciliary muscle, i.e., tonic accommodation. The choroidal tension was therefore dependent upon the ciliary muscle tonus. The tension of the choroid, in turn, determined its direct ability to resist the forces of the normal intraocular pressure and its subsequent effect on the sclera, and ultimately axial length. Hence, the ability of the globe to resist such stretching forces was directly related to the tonus of the ciliary muscle/choroid complex. The greater the tonus, i.e., the higher the tonic accommodation, the greater the resistance to any such internal forces. Consequently, the less will be any posterior pole expansion, and accordingly, any axial-induced myopia. Conversely, the presence of reduced ciliary tonicity, i.e., the lower the tonic accommodation, and hence concurrently low choroidal tension, would pose little resistance to the internal forces from the intraocular pressure. As a consequence, this tension would be transmitted to the sclera and predispose it to stretching, thus resulting in greater posterior pole expansion and therefore an increase in axial-based myopia.

Investigations on tonic accommodation as a function of refractive state of the eye have yielded some results in support with the aforementioned theory (See Chapter 2 for a detailed discussion). While the findings have been equivocal, nonetheless, just over half of the studies (53%) have demonstrated that myopes had reduced tonic accommodation relative to the other refractive groups (see Table 2-7a). Hence, myopic eyes which presumably exhibited relatively low tonic accommodation values may be less resistant to the forces exerted by the intraocular pressure, and thus be more vulnerable to axial elongation, according to Van Alphen's theory. This latter notion is also consistent with the vast majority of reports showing a correlation between axial length and a myopic refractive state.

Accommodative Adaptation

Since nearwork has been implicated as a potential etiological factor of myopia, and in a further attempt to investigate the role of tonic accommodation in the myopization process, studies have been directed to determine the effect of near work on tonic accommodation (see Table 2-8). Several studies reported transient myopic "shifts" in tonic accommodation following a sustained period of near vision. It was postulated that the observed accommodative hysteresis/accommodative adaptation phenomenon served as a precursor to axial myopia (Ebenholtz 1983), the precise mechanism of which was not specified. Repeated periods of near vision without total decay of accommodative adaptation might potentially transform these transient myopic changes into a more permanent form of myopia (Gilmartin and Bullimore 1991, Rosenfield et al. 1992a). Furthermore, it was proposed that these transient changes in so-called "post-task tonic accommodation" represented actual modification of the tonic innervation to the ciliary muscle per se (Owens 1991).

These apparent post-task shifts in tonic accommodation, which actually reflected blur-driven accommodative adaptation (Figure 4-8) *and not* tonic accommodation per se (Hung 1992), were found to be inversely related to tonic accommodation (Ebenholtz 1985, Owens and Wolf-Kelly 1987, Morse and Smith 1993). That is, individuals with higher levels of tonic accommodation exhibited reduced accommodative adaptation effects, and conversely, those with lower levels of tonic accommodation demonstrated enhanced accommodative adaptation. Furthermore, Owens and Wolf-Kelly (1987) found that individuals in whom tonic accommodation was less than 1D showed the greatest accommodative adaptation, whereas those in whom tonic accommodation was between 1 to 2 D exhibited the least; those with values of 2D or higher fell in between. In addition, it was also reported that the time course of decay of accommodative adaptation was related to the pre-task level of tonic accommodation (Gilmartin and Bullimore 1987). A faster decay was demonstrated for individuals exhibiting a pre-task tonic accommodative level greater than 0.55D, while a slower decay characterized by an absence of a hyperopic shift was found for individuals with tonic accommodation less than 0.55D. Based on the foregoing, and given the general finding of lower tonic accommodation found for myopes, *one would predict greater accommodative adaptation with a protracted decay in the myopes.* In fact, there is some evidence to suggest that accommodative adaptation effects may indeed be increased and prolonged in myopes (see Table 2-8). However, this was not a consistent finding. For example, there were other studies which demonstrated that accommodative adaptation was invariant with refractive group (see Table 2-8). Once again, some inconsistency may not be unexpected with an effect that is small and transient.

The difference in tonic accommodation and accommodative adaptation found between refractive groups can perhaps be accounted for by differences in autonomic innervation. Extant pharmacological evidence has indicated that tonic accommodation is primarily parasympathetically-mediated, and, furthermore, that intersubject variability in tonic accommodation is a consequence of variation in parasympathetic innervation to the ciliary muscle among different individuals (Gilmartin and Hogan 1985a). Hence, the lower tonic accommodation found in many myopes is probably reflective of reduced parasympathetic innervation. In fact, it was previously suggested by McBrien and Millodot (1988) that myopes exhibited reduced parasympathetic innervation (See Chapter 2). What are the implications of such a presumed attenuated input from the parasympathetic nervous system? Since the magnitude of sympathetic innervation is dependent on the concurrent level of parasympathetic innervation (Tornqvist 1967), individuals who exhibit reduced parasympathetic innervation would therefore also have reduced sympathetic innervation. Work in this area has in fact revealed that late-onset myopes in particular may be characterized by deficient sympathetic innervation (Gilmartin and Bullimore, 1991, Rosenfield and Gilmartin 1989), although there is still some question (Gilmartin and Winfield, 1995). Since a function of the sympathetic input is to inhibit or attenuate accommodative adaptation (Ebenholtz 1985, Gilmartin and Hogan 1985b, Gilmartin and Bullimore 1987, Gilmartin et al. 1992), then a deficit in sympathetic innervation would predispose these individuals to manifest a greater degree of accommodative adaptation. Thus, the increased adaptation found in many myopes is indeed predicted for the aforementioned reason. In addition, a protracted baseline regression pattern to pre-task tonic levels was also reported in myopes (Fisher et al. 1987, Rosenfield and Gilmartin 1988a, Gilmartin et al. 1989a, 1989b, Gilmartin and Bullimore 1991, Strang et al. 1994). Once again, the slower baseline decay or regression rate characterizing myopes is consistent with and lends credence to the notion of a deficit in their sympathetic input. The longer decay time constant also implicates the potential role of abnormal accommodative adaptation (Ebenholtz 1983) and its related pharmacology in the etiology of myopia.

However, several points need to be addressed. Although many studies have shown that myopes exhibit reduced tonic accommodation relative to emmetropes, this reduction is probably not of sufficient magnitude to support Van Alphen's theory, at least in any direct manner. For example, the mean tonic accommodation in emmetropes was 1.16D, while myopes exhibited a mean value of 0.83D (see Table 2-7a). This 0.33D difference in tonus of the ciliary muscle probably does not pose a substantially different resistance to the forces of intraocular pressure. For example, the maximal force of contraction of isolated human ciliary muscle was reported to be approximately 0.5g (Suzuki 1983, Lograno and Reibaldi 1986). Assuming that this maximum force is required to produce a 15D total accommodative amplitude response in a young individual, and further that this relationship is probably reasonably linear and invariant with age for teenagers and young adults, then the 0.33D mean difference in tonic accommodation between myopes and emmetropes would yield a proportional and differential force equivalent to 0.011g. This difference in force between the two refractive groups represents only 2% of the maximum total force. Furthermore, this value and its potential impact become reduced dramatically if we consider the differential forces in play during normal viewing conditions. The contribution of tonic accommodation and hence its impact to the aggregate accommodative response under normal binocular closed-loop viewing conditions is considerably smaller. According to the Hung and Semmlow (1980) dual-interactive model of accommodation and vergence, the contribution of tonic accommodation (TA) to the overall accommodative response is equivalent to TA * (1/1+ACG), where ACG= the accommodative controller gain. Assuming an ACG of 9 (Mordi 1991, Ong et al. 1993), the component contribution of tonic accommodation to the overall steady-state accommodative response would not exceed 10% of its value. Taking the 0.33D difference in tonic accommodation into account, it means that this effective value under closed-loop conditions is actually equivalent to 0.033D, which is only 0.2% of the maximal potential myodioptric force of the ciliary muscle. It is doubtful that such a small difference, even over a considerable period of time, i.e., months or even years, could have significant physiological and anatomical impact. In addition, more recent studies using open-field infrared instrumentation, which essentially eliminated proximal influences, reported even lower mean values of tonic accommodation (Rosenfield et al. 1993). This would further reduce the absolute differential values found between refractive groups, and hence any potential impact on scleral stretching and axial myopia.

In addition to the above argument, not all studies found reduced tonic accommodation in myopes. Forty-seven percent failed to demonstrate this trend. While 38% reported no differences between groups (see Table 2-7c), 9% even showed the reverse trend (see Table 2-7b). This lack of consistency in findings suggests that the proposed role of tonic accommodation in the etiology of myopia, if any, is not a very potent one. Furthermore, preliminary longitudinal studies do not fully support the finding of differential tonic accommodation as a function of refraction. While Owens et al. (1989) noted correlated group changes between tonic accommodation and distance refraction over a two-to four-year period, nonetheless such changes were not correlated *within* many individual subjects. Thus, the group effect was in fact misleading.

Although there is ample and consistent evidence relating near work and accommodative adaptation, the role of the latter as an etiological factor in myopia has not been fully understood. It has been suggested that these accommodative adaptation effects were due to an actual change in the innervation to ciliary muscle (Owens 1991). However, this is an incorrect interpretation as mentioned earlier. Tonic accommodation per se represents baseline neurology of probable midbrain origin, and thus is not that readily and rapidly modifiable. In fact, it has been shown to be relatively stable over both the short- and long-term (see Rosenfield et al. 1993 for a review). Certainly, simply focusing on letters for a few minutes should have little impact on midbrain activity. If accommodative hysteresis in fact represented an altered tonic input, then based on Van Alphen's theory (1961), such myopic shifts in tonic accommodation would in fact *inhibit* the development of myopia. The nearwork-induced myopic changes with accommodative adaptation would presumably reflect enhanced or increased ciliary muscle tonus. This translates into an overall transient increase in tonicity of the choroid. According to Van Alphen, this is synonymous with an increase in choroidal resistance to intraocular pressure which subsequently translates into a greater resistance to scleral stretch, and accordingly inhibition of any axially-induced myopia from developing. However, see Chapter 5.

Nearwork-Induced Transient Myopia

Instead of representing a true change in tonic innervation, the post-task accommodative change appears to reflect the slow accommodative adaptive neural component (Hung 1992), and hence accommodative adaptation/hysteresis (Figure 4-8). As gleaned from numerous studies, it appears that accommodative adaptation effects are generalizable over a wide range of conditions. Following a sustained near vision task, accommodative adaptation effects occur and can be measured under both open- and closed-loop viewing conditions. More specifically, the accommodative hysteresis measurements found in the dark by several investigators represent the accommodative adaptation effects superimposed on the relatively stable baseline tonic accommodation level, and these adaptive effects only become fully manifested under open-loop conditions. The effects of accommodative adaptation may in part also be manifested transiently under closed-loop

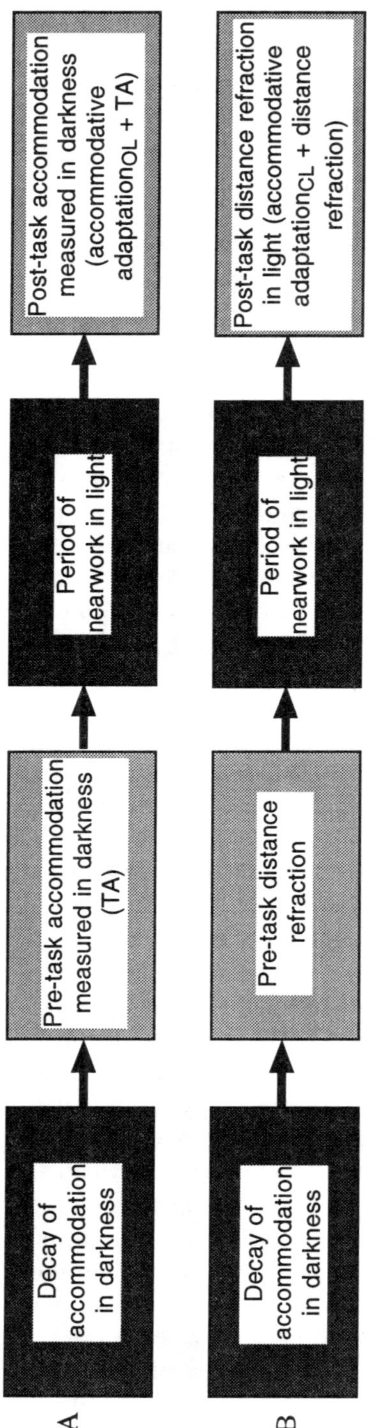

Figure 4-9: Diagram distinguishing the experimental paradigm used in (A) the assessment of accommodative adaptation (open-loop accommodative adaptation) and (B) nearwork-induced transient myopia (closed-loop accommodative adaptation); TA= tonic accommodation, OL= open-loop, CL= closed-loop.

conditions as well, such as is evidenced in the biased post-task closed-loop near point of accommodation value (Fisher et al. 1987), post-task intermediate test distances (Takahashi 1983), and post-task accommodative stimulus/response function (Owens and Wolf-Kelly 1987). Hence, the accommodative adaptation effects manifested in the presence of blur feedback and measured under closed-loop conditions are regarded as being superimposed on the distance refraction, and hence are regarded to be transient ("pseudo")myopia (Figure 4-9). Extant literature has documented transient myopic changes in the post-task distance refraction following a period of near vision under a variety of natural and experimental closed-loop paradigms using various criteria as described earlier in this chapter. This phenomenon has become more commonly known as nearwork-induced transient myopia (NITM). The transient myopic changes in normal individuals were typically small with a mean of 0.33D and a range from 0.12 to 1.30D. These effects were generally less than those recorded under open-loop conditions in similar groups. This can be explained by the fact that under closed-loop conditions, the effective damping action of visual feedback suppresses the full magnitude of accommodative adaptation from being manifested, with the limiting factor being the depth-of-focus of the eye. In the attempt to relate accommodative adaptation to permanent myopia, studying transient myopia in the light rather than accommodative adaptation in the dark therefore seems more logical and relevant. With transient myopia, both the inducing and measuring periods were obtained under conditions of normal visual feedback and hence simulated naturalistic conditions. On the other hand, the phenomenon of accommodative adaptation/hysteresis, which was typically measured under open-loop conditions in the dark, was clearly not naturalistic. It would therefore not be an optimal approach, since these open-loop accommodative adaptation effects may not translate directly and in all its entirety to the naturalistic closed-loop illuminated viewing conditions.

POSSIBLE MECHANISMS OF NITM

What mechanisms may be responsible for inducing NITM? Since the various near visual tasks involved accommodation and vergence (in some cases), one should first distinguish the contribution of each. Studies cited earlier have demonstrated NITM under monocular conditions. Moreover, recent investigations by Ong et al. (1994, 1996) and Ong (1996) have ruled out any major contribution from vergence and vergence-accommodation and rather have implicated blur-driven accommodation as being the predominant factor for inducing NITM. Therefore, to address the question appropriately, one should first investigate the possible mechanisms involved in the process of blur-driven accommodation.

The ocular components that have been implicated to vary as a function of blur-driven accommodation are axial length and the ciliary body-crystalline lens apparatus.

1) Axial length: Investigations regarding accommodatively-induced axial length changes appear at first glance to be equivocal (Young 1801, Coleman et al. 1969, Storey and Rabie 1983, Beauchamp and Mitchell 1985, Lepper and Trier 1987, Soriano 1987, Shum et al. 1993). A review of the literature has demonstrated mean changes ranging from a *decrease* of 0.08mm to an increase of 0.10mm (Coleman et al. 1969, Storey and Rabie 1983, Beauchamp and Mitchell 1985, Lepper and Trier 1987, Soriano 1987, Shum et al. 1993), which translates to approximately only ±0.30D, but which in fact equals the average magnitude of NITM. However, if axial length changes were a general mechanism in the accommodative process and NITM, one would expect to measure only *increases* in axial length. Thus, in all probability, and in agreement with one's intuition, no real changes in axial length occurred with accommodation, and the reported

apparent bidirectional changes simply represent biological and instrumentation noise in the measurements.

2) Ciliary muscle-crystalline lens apparatus:

(a) Anatomical: A minority of investigators have implicated the lens as the mechanism responsible for producing environmentally-induced myopia (Sato 1957, Goldschmidt 1968). However, they failed to present irrefutable evidence in support of their theories, which were generally vague and non-specific. Nonetheless, a brief discussion of these theories is still warranted. Although they relate to more permanent forms of myopia, the same mechanisms can also be applied towards transient forms of myopia. In Goldschmidt's monograph (1968), he indicated that the etiologic mechanism was an increase in lens power rather than an elongation of axial length. His rationale was that as the lens continued to grow throughout life, its refractive power was constantly being modified, and as it developed, the lens was therefore susceptible to environmental influences. Likewise, the refractive theory of Sato (1957) postulated that the physiological adaptive function was related to the refractive power of the lens. Sustained near work and therefore a continuous state of increased accommodation lead to involuntary contraction due to the increased tonus of the ciliary muscle that could not be relaxed, and this eventually resulted in so-called "organic" changes in the lens and ciliary apparatus. More specifically, Sato cited changes in the intra- and extra-capsular components of the crystalline lens, in its refractive index and elasticity, the ciliary muscle, the zonules of Zinn, and even the vitreous humor. A large part of Sato's theory depended on the elastic properties of the crystalline lens. An investigation in this area (Kikkawa and Sato 1963) showed that the sustained application of external compressive forces on the lens resulted in plastic or permanent deformation following the removal of that force. An elastic aftereffect was evident, but recovery was slow and incomplete. However, the study was conducted under unnatural and extreme conditions. Forces with magnitudes ranging from 0.7g to 2.2g were used. These magnitudes were considerably greater than those occurring during the normal maximum accommodative response (~0.5g) (Suzuki 1983, Lograno and Reibaldi 1986). In addition, since these specimens consisted of rabbit and cat eyes, the same findings may not apply directly to humans, as accommodative ability has been demonstrated to be species-dependent (van Alphen 1976, Suzuki 1983). At first glance, the lenticular/ciliary body theories of Goldschmidt (1968) and of Sato (1957) could, at best, only account for a small portion of the myopia, as most myopias clearly have a major axial length correlated component (Stenstrom 1948, van Alphen 1961, Curtin 1985, McBrien and Millodot 1987). However, this does not rule out the possibility that an initial spasm-like lens/ciliary muscle-based myopia could cause retinal defocus of sufficient amount to stimulate axial length growth. This notion awaits careful investigation. See more detailed discussions in Chapters 4, 6 and 7.

More recently, an investigation by Ong et al. (1994) presented data that would be inconsistent with the notion of a simple biomechanically-induced lenticular hysteresis. In this study, while the within-task accommodative responses to different conditions were approximately equivalent, the NITM was not. This implied that the lens biomechanics and ciliary muscle force for the different conditions were also approximately equivalent. However, the initial post-task NITM amplitude, as well as the time course of decay for these conditions, were significantly different. Therefore, the task-induced adaptation may not relate directly to the total amount of accommodation exerted nor to the lens/capsule biomechanics and its related ciliary muscle forces per se, but rather to the blur-driven component only. Although it is highly unlikely that the biomechanics and forces played any substantial role in inducing NITM, nonetheless, they may still be involved in the development of environmentally-induced myopia.

(b) Neurological: It is possible that a sustained near visual task may induce a change at the neurological level, such as increased duration and/or frequency of spike potentials, which may lead to a prolonged response decay pattern, i.e., neuromuscular hysteresis, following the removal of stimulation. However, the work by Suzuki (1983) seemed to indicate otherwise. In this study, electrical stimulation of exposed ciliary nerves of isolated ciliary muscle strips from bovine eyes evoked twitch-like contractions. An increase in either stimulus duration or frequency resulted in an increased response magnitude, but without change in its time course of decay upon cessation of stimulation. Baseline was generally attained in approximately 4 to 5 seconds. Prolonged contraction as well as protracted decay (5 to 6 minutes) were only observed when a parasympathomimetic agent such as physostigmine was added. From this, Suzuki concluded that the ciliary muscle contraction was not directly neurologically mediated via electric potentials, but rather neuropharmacologically through the action of neurotransmitters of the autonomic nervous system.

(c) Pharmacological: At the receptor level, it has been well-documented that the accommodative system receives dual innervation from the autonomic nervous system, consisting primarily of a parasympathetic (cholinergic) and secondarily a sympathetic (adrenergic) component (Gilmartin 1986). The former division is characterized by a rapid onset of action with its response completed in 1 second or so (Campbell and Westheimer 1960). An increase or decrease in parasympathetic stimulation resulted in an increase and decrease in accommodation, respectively (Biggs et al. 1959, Tornqvist 1967). On the other hand, the sympathetic division is characterized by a slow temporal course, with a response time of 10 to 40 seconds

(Tornqvist 1967, Rosenfield and Gilmartin 1989). Its magnitude, which is directly related to the concurrent level of background parasympathetic activity, is generally small, and its action is inhibitory (i.e., "negative" accommodation) in nature. Following the completion of a sustained accommodative task, the relatively long sympathetic decay is reflected motorically as accommodative adaptation and in part as NITM. Due to its slow time course, it is proposed that the function of the sympathetic system primarily involves sustained visual tasks, and more specifically, attenuation of the magnitude and duration of the post-task transient myopic adaptive changes (Gilmartin and Bullimore 1987). It is therefore conceivable that a deficit in this inhibitory sympathetic innervation would result in a larger accommodative aftereffect, including a greater magnitude and slower decay of transient myopia (Rosenfield et al. 1992a, 1992b, Gilmartin and Bullimore 1987). This is an area for further clinical investigation, especially with respect to preventive and developmental aspects of myopia in children, assuming transient myopia may either be directly or indirectly involved in the development of permanent axially-based myopia.

NEARWORK-INDUCED TRANSIENT MYOPIA, ACCOMMODATIVE SPASM, PSEUDOMYOPIA, AND PERMANENT MYOPIA

Nearwork-Induced Transient Myopia

The phenomenon of NITM is lenticular in origin. These lenticular changes reflect a hysteresis phenomenon or "accommodative aftereffect" (i.e., a system response may be affected by its immediate past history) of the accommodative system, which is a normal physiological response. This is analogous to the vergence system's "fusional aftereffect" or vergence adaptation/hysteresis that may be present immediately following vergence range testing (Borish 1970). Accommodative hysteresis and NITM may involve both a central higher-level innervational and blur computational component, and a peripheral lower-level neuromuscular innervational component.

Accommodative Spasm

A grossly abnormal extension of this "lower-level" ciliary muscle hysteresis is the clinical phenomenon of "accommodative or ciliary spasm." The available literature on ciliary spasm defines it as being an excessive, unnecessary and inappropriate contraction of the ciliary muscle (Borish 1970, Michaels 1980). It can be drug-induced, e.g., following instillation of parasympathomimetics or anticholinesterases, or disease-induced, e.g., following iritis, corneal disease, episcleritis, lesions of the trigeminal nerve, etc. (Michaels 1980, Goldstein and Schneekloth 1996). These "pathological" or drug-related kinds of accommodative spasms must be differentiated from the "functional" or non-pathological accommodative spasm that is of interest here and which occurs in some younger patients as a consequence of prolonged near visual work (Duke-Elder and Abrams 1970, Grosvenor 1989). This functional type of spasm is traditionally reported to result from apparent muscular "fatigue" (Duke-Elder and Abrams 1970) or excessive accommodative effort. Accommodative spasm, in general clinical terms, is attributed to excessive ciliary muscle tonus of parasympathetic origin (Duke-Elder and Abrams 1970). Once the spastic ciliary muscle exhibits such "hypertonicity," it is prevented from fully relaxing during attempted changes in focus from near to distant objects (Grosvenor 1989). As a consequence, resultant symptoms may include distance and near blurred vision, headache, photophobia, diplopia, reduced amplitude, and miosis (Michaels 1980).

Although nearwork-induced transient myopia and accommodative spasm possess several aspects common to both, as they are lenticular in origin and involve an inability to relax accommodation at far, nonetheless, there are also clear differences that cannot be ignored. First, the asymptomatic type of nearwork-induced transient myopia is normal. It dissipates quickly, within a matter of seconds, or minutes in the worst case scenario. Second, such NITM is small in magnitude. And, third, it is likely to involve both the central and peripheral neural adaptational components. On the other hand, accommodative spasm represents an abnormal clinically-defined entity with pronounced symptoms. First, it is relatively fixed at a certain near accommodative level, so that efforts to change accommodation in either direction are typically futile or at best difficult. Second, it is generally larger in magnitude (a few diopters). And third, it is also likely to be purely of a lower order or more peripheral nature.

An overall conceptual scheme for the relation between the two is made by considering accommodative responsivity along a continuum (Figure 4-10). At one extreme end lies the normal dynamic accommodative re-

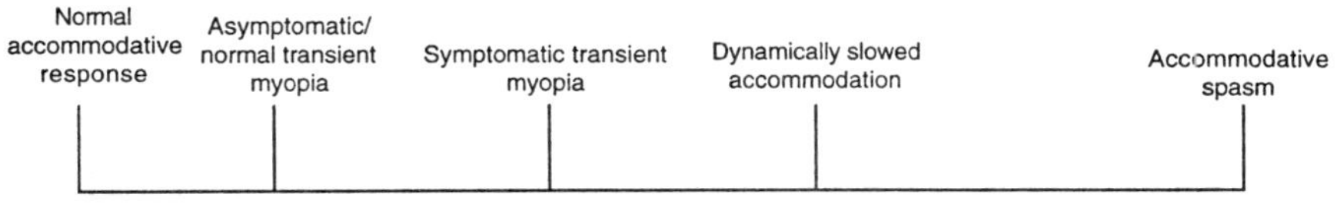

Figure 4-10 : Relation between various accommodative response types.

sponse. This is the response reported following brief near tasks and is characterized by a change of accommodation in either direction being completed within a second or so (Campbell and Westheimer 1960). Adjacent to the normal dynamic response along the continuum is the phenomenon of normal asymptomatic transient myopia (Rosenfield et al. 1992a, Ong and Ciuffreda, 1995). Yet, further along is found a more exaggerated form of transient myopia exhibited by symptomatic individuals (Ciuffreda and Ordoñez 1995). In this scenario, the abnormal responses are either greater in magnitude, slower in recovery/decay, and/or more variable than found in normal NITM. Furthermore, these individuals report blur for several seconds or more at distance following nearwork. And at the other end of the continuum is found the overall dynamically-slowed response (Liu et al. 1979), and finally abnormal accommodative spasm, which may represent a grossly aberrant form of transient myopia. And, in this last case, blur is an even more persistent and troublesome symptom.

Pseudomyopia

It is frequently indicated in the literature that the abnormal state of accommodative spasm associated with near work may become intransigent in pseudomyopia. Pseudomyopia is a reversible form of myopia, resulting from spasm of accommodation (Borish 1970, Michaels 1980, Grosvenor 1989). Consequently, emmetropes and hyperopes may appear to be myopes, and myopes may appear to be more myopic, under non-cycloplegic clinical examination. Pseudomyopes experience frequent symptomatic episodes during near work (Michaels 1980). They also typically report transitory blurred distant vision following an extended period of near work (Grosvenor 1989). Thus, several descriptive terms such as school myopia, false myopia, functional myopia, or refractive myopia have been coined to represent the same abnormal condition (Borish 1970). However, both frank accommodative spasm and pseudomyopia of a functional nature have been traditionally believed to be relatively rare, certainly much less frequent than general accommodative dysfunction (Goldstein and Schneekloth 1996).

But not all would agree with these conventional and conservative notions. Several investigations have suggested an association between a continuous state of ciliary spasm resulting from sustained accommodation and nearwork-induced acquired myopia. The ciliary spasm and consequent pseudomyopia were proposed to progress into permanent myopia. Sato (1957), being its most ardent proponent, indicated that a prolonged and fixed accommodative state lead to organic changes, e.g., hypertrophy of the ciliary muscle and eventually lenticular changes. Similarly, Eggers (1963) postulated that overaccommodation gave rise to increased tonicity of the ciliary apparatus, which resulted in a permanent change in both the ciliary

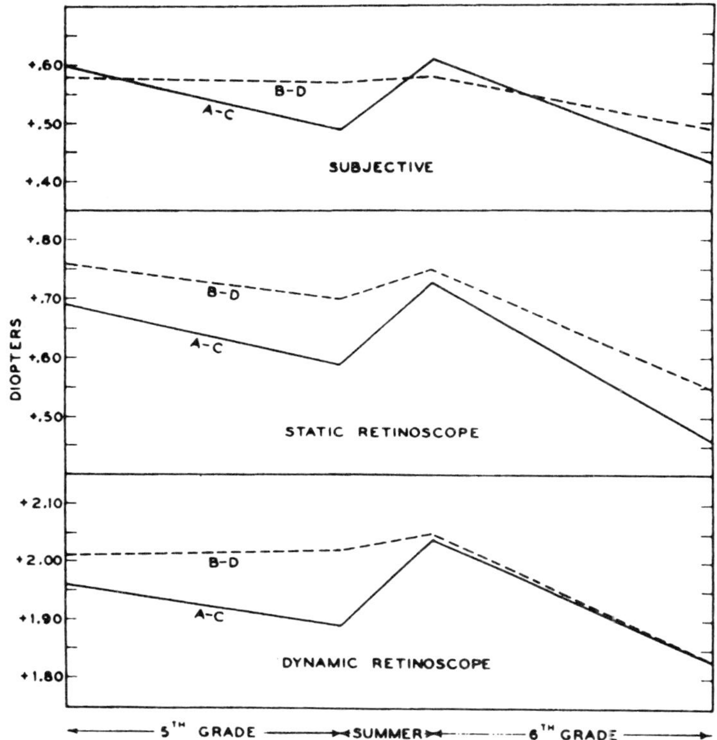

Figure 4-11 : The average spherical corrections for the pupils in the experimental (A-C) and control (B-D) rooms are indicated by the solid and broken-lines, respectively (Reprinted with permission, Luckiesh and Moss 1939).

body and the crystalline lens. Increased ciliary tonicity was also espoused by Holm (1926) and later by Luckiesh and Moss (1939) and Owens and Harris (1980). In the latter two studies, myopic refractive shifts were noted during the school year, while hyperopic shifts were reported during the summer months, suggesting the occurrence of pseudomyopic changes during the school year (Figure 4-11). Finally, Goldschmidt (1968), who proposed a similar mechanism, suggested that it was more readily applied to late-onset myopes, although it could develop in early-onset myopes as well in conjunction with the genetically-based component of their myopia. Goldschmidt speculated that this type of myopia was probably due to an increase in lens power rather than axial elongation, with the rationale being that the lens continued to grow throughout life and was therefore susceptible to external influences. In all of these studies, their hypotheses hinged on a myopia that was lenticular-based and thus purely refractive in nature.

However, there was little direct evident to support these interesting, and for the time, somewhat intuitively satisfying, speculations.

Other investigators have also proposed a transitional phase between lenticular myopia and permanent axially-based myopia. More specifically, they suggested that lens-based refractive changes acted as a precursor to axial myopia. As early as 1883, Cohn (1883) proposed that sustained accommodation due to near activity resulted in an "accommodation cramp or spasm." This sustained ciliary muscle contraction led to increased convexity of the lens which in turn gave rise to "lens-myopia" when individuals then attempted to focus into the distance. Following prolonged nearwork, the ciliary muscle was not capable of recovering sufficiently, hence the "transient lens-myopia gradually passes into the chronic axis-myopia". Unfortunately, the precise mechanism for this critical transition was not elucidated. More recently, Mei and Rong (1994) proposed a similar two-stage process in schoolchildren. The initial stage consisted of a lenticular-based pseudomyopia resulting from prolonged accommodation at near. This was followed by the onset of permanent myopia of axial length in origin. In their longitudinal investigation of Chinese schoolchildren aged 9-12 years, 64 out of the 194 eyes developed myopia in the course of 2 years. In its early stages, an unusually high prevalence of pseudomyopia (36%) based on cycloplegic refraction results was noted for those who became myopic, although the pseudomyopia was, in almost all cases, shortlived. Within 6 months to a year of reexamination, it was found that most of the reported cases of pseudomyopia had progressed to permanent myopia. Their concurrent biometric data indicated that the corresponding changes at this second stage involved only lengthening of the vitreous chamber depth and thus overall axial length. No changes were found in either anterior chamber depth or lens thickness. Once again, the precise mechanism remains unknown. However, as discussed in several sections of this book, retinal defocus may in fact act as a trigger mechanism for myopic axial alongation.

Permanent Myopia

Findings from the preceding two studies would contradict to some extent the notion of purely lenticular changes and the related simple refractive myopia introduced by other investigators such as Sato and Goldschmidt. In fact, work on the biometrics of the eye as related to overall refraction does not support any *permanent* lens-based component in the myopization process. By all accounts, the crystalline lens in myopes is actually reported to be generally *flatter* and *reduced* in power relative to emmetropes and hyperopes (Tron 1929, Stenstrom 1946, 1947, 1948, Sato 1957, Franceschetti and Gernet 1965, Franceschetti and Luyckx 1966, Francois and Goes 1969, Gernet 1981, Garner et al. 1992). Furthermore, there is no clinical evidence to suggest histological changes in the ciliary muscle of young myopes. Studies have revealed that the primary factor responsible for myopic development was axial elongation (Stenstrom 1948, Van Alphen 1961, Grosvenor and Scott 1993). In particular, late-onset myopia is reported to be predominantly axial in nature (McBrien and Millodot 1987, Fledelius 1995). *However,* it is possible that these investigators might have missed this potentially important "transitional phase" lens-based pseudomyopia in a subgroup of children who then go on to develop permanent myopia (Mei and Rong 1994).

Clearly, this interesting and potentially important finding warrants further investigation. First, it should be replicated in various clinical populations. For example, is there an upper age limit for the phenomenon? Are certain subgroups most susceptible? If so, why? And, second, if this is found to be true, clinicians should use such information to begin to develop aggressive clinical protocols which at a minimum would monitor and advise such children and their parents, and ideally would reverse or even prevent the condition from becoming manifest in the first place. In addition to frequent and careful manifest and cycloplegic refractive measurements, incorporating objective autorefraction and clinical ultrasonic assessments, aggressive prevention and/or intervention should be instituted which may involve drug therapy, oculomotor vision therapy (especially involving accommodative facility exercises), visualization and relaxation techniques, auditory and visual biofeedback, high powered bifocal lenses, frequent rest periods during nearwork activity, and/or changes in the ergonomics of the schools and work environment to counteract any pseudomyopic precursor component.

SUMMARY

In this chapter, the literature on nearwork-induced transient myopia (NITM) is reviewed, with NITM being defined as the short-term pseudomyopic far point shift immediately following a sustained near visual task. A majority of these investigations demonstrated the presence of NITM for a variety of test parameters, e.g., visual acuity, contrast sensitivity and far point change. While the precise etiology and implications of NITM remain unclear, speculations regarding its origin and relevance to clinical myopia are discussed.

APPENDIX 1

TABLE 4-3: COMPONENT CONTRIBUTION PER THE COMPREHENSIVE ACCOMMODATIVE AND VERGENCE STATIC MODEL

VIEWING CONDITION	NITM (D)	COMPOSITE ACCOMMO-DATIVE RESPONSE (D)	BLUR COMPONENT (D)	VERGENCE COMPONENT (D)	PROXIMAL COMPONENT (D)	TONIC COMPONENT (D)
(1) Far/ Congruent	0.08	0.22	0.146	0.008	0.006	0.062
(2) Far/ -2.50D Lens	0.39	2.27	2.190	0.008	0.006	0.062
(3) Far/BO Prisms	0.05	0.33	0.146	0.114	0.006	0.062
(4) Far/ -2.50 D Lens & BO Prisms	0.27	2.37	2.190	0.114	0.006	0.062
(5) Far/ Monocular/ Pinhole	0.10	0.69	NSD	NSD	0.075	0.610
(6) Near/ Congruent	0.21	2.46	2.190	0.114	0.100	0.062
(7) Near/ +2.50 D Lens	-0.06	0.27	0	0.114	0.100	0.062
(8) Near/ BI Prisms	0.30	2.35	2.190	0	0.100	0.062
(9) Near/ +2.50 D Lens & BI Prisms	0.06	0.16	0	0	0.100	0.062
(10) Near/ Monocular/ Pinhole	0.18	1.74	NSD	NSD	1.130	0.610
(11) Near/ Monocular	0.21	2.43	2.270	NSD	0.100	0.055
(12) Near/ Non-compen-satible Blur	0.33	*	*	0.114	0.100	0.062

Table Legend: NITM= nearwork-induced transient myopia, D= diopters, BO= base-out, BI= base-in, *= cannot be calculated, and NSD = not stimulus driven. See model Figure 4-8.

To solve for the overall accommodative response for conditions #1through #4, and #6 through #9 (Hung et al., 1996), where $AR_{Acl,\ Vcl}$ = accommodative response under dual closed-loop conditions:

$AR_{Acl,Vcl}$= {[ACG * (1+VCG) - ACG * VCG * AC * CA] * AS + VCG * CA * VS + [APG * (1+VCG) - APG * VCG * AC * CA + VPG * CA] * PDG * DS + (1+VCG) * ABIAS - VCG * CA * VBIAS} / {(1+ACG) * (1+VCG) - ACG * VCG * AC * CA} (1)

To solve for the overall accommodative response for conditions #5 and #10; where $AR_{Aol,Vol}$ = accommodative response under dual open-loop conditions:

$AR_{Aol,Vol}$= (APG + VPG * CA) * PDG * DS + ABIAS (2)

To solve for the overall accommodative response for condition #11, where $AR_{Acl,Vol}$ = accommodative response with vergence open-loop:

$AR_{Acl,Vol}$= [ACG/ (1+ACG)] * AS + [1/ (1+ACG)] * (APG + VPG * CA) * PDG * DS + (1/ 1+ACG) * ABIAS (3)

To solve for the individual accommodative components:

Blur-driven component= {[ACG * (1+VCG) - ACG * VCG * AC * CA] * AS }/ [(1+ACG) * (1+VCG) - ACG * VCG * AC * CA] (4)

Disparity vergence component = [VCG * CA * VS] / [(1+ACG) * (1+VCG) - ACG * VCG * AC * CA] (5)

Proximal component = {[APG * (1+VCG) - APG * VCG * AC * CA + VPG * CA] * PDG * DS] / [(1+ACG) * (1+VCG) - ACG * VCG * AC * CA] (6)

Tonic component = [(1+VCG) * ABIAS - VCG * CA * VBIAS] / [(1+ACG) * (1+VCG) - ACG * VCG * AC * CA] (7)

The model parameter values as well as the legend for the abbreviations are as follows:

Accommodative controller gain (ACG)	10.0
Vergence controller gain (VCG)	150.0
Accommodative convergence (AC)	0.80 MA/D
Convergence accommodation (CA)	0.37 D/MA
Perceived distance gain (PDG)	0.212
Accommodative proximal gain (APG)	2.100
Vergence proximal gain (VPG)	0.067
Tonic accommodation (ABIAS)	0.61D
Tonic vergence (VBIAS)	0.29 MA

REFERENCES

Ball GV. Symptoms in eye examination. London: Butterworth Scientific; 1982: 52.

Beauchamp R, Mitchell B. Ultrasound measures of vitreous chamber depth during ocular accommodation. Am J Optom Physiol Opt. 1985; 62: 523-32.

Biggs RD, Alpern M, Bennett DR. The effect of sympathomimetic drugs upon the amplitude of accommodation. Am J Ophthalmol. 1959; 48: 169-72.

Blustein GH, Rosenfield M, Ciuffreda KJ. Does dark accommodation really change following sustained near fixation? Optom Vis Sci (Suppl). 1993; 70: 16.

Borish IM. Clinical Refraction, 3rd ed. Chicago: The Professional Press, Inc.; 1970.

Campbell FW, Westheimer G. Dynamics of accommodation responses of the human eye. J Physiol. 1960; 151: 285-95.

Ciuffreda KJ. Accommodation and its anomalies. In: Charman WN, ed. Vision and Visual Dysfunction, vol. 1. London: MacMillan; 1991: 231-79.

Ciuffreda KJ. Accommodation, pupil and presbyopia. In: Borish IM, Benjamin J, eds. Clinical Refraction:Principles and Practice. Philadelphia: Saunders; in press.

Ciuffreda KJ, Colburn C, Wallis D. Effect of stimulus duration and dioptric demand on transient myopia. Invest Ophthalmol Vis Sci (Suppl). 1996; 37: 164.

Ciuffreda KJ, Ordoñez X. Abnormal transient myopia in symptomatic individuals after sustained nearwork. Optom Vis Sci. 1995; 72: 506-10.

Cohn H. Hygiene of the eye in schools. trans. Turnbull WP. London: Simpkin, Marshall & Co.; 1883.

Coleman J, Wuchinich D, Carlin B. Accommodative changes in the axial dimension of the human eye. In: Gitter KA, Keeney AH, Sarin LK, Meyer D, eds. Ophthalmic Ultrasound. St. Louis: C.V. Mosby Co.; 1969: 134-41.

Curtin BJ. The Myopias- basic science and clinical management. Philadelphia: Harper & Row; 1985.

Dainoff MJ, Happ A. Visual fatigue and occupational stress in VDT operators. Human Factors. 1981; 23: 421-38.

Duke-Elder S, Abrams D. System of Ophthalmology, vol. V. Ophthalmic Optics and Refraction. St. Louis: C.V. Mosby Co.; 1970, 469-74.

Ebenholtz SM. Accommodative hysteresis: a precursor for induced myopia? Invest Ophthalmol Vis Sci. 1983; 24: 513-5.

Ebenholtz SM. Accommodative hysteresis: relation to resting focus. Am J Optom Physiol Opt. 1985; 62: 755-62.

Ebenholtz SM, Zander PAL. Accommodative hysteresis: influence on closed loop measures of far point and near point. Invest Ophthalmol Vis Sci. 1987; 28: 1246-9.

Eggers H. The causes and treatment of school myopia. Eye, Ear, Nose and Throat Monthly. 1963; 42: 50-55.

Ehrlich DL. Near vision stress: Vergence adaptation and accommodative fatigue. Ophthal Physiol Opt. 1987; 7: 353-7.

Fisher SK, Ciuffreda KJ, Levine S. Tonic accommodation, accommodative hysteresis, and refractive error. Am J Optom Physiol Opt. 1987; 64: 799-809.

Fledelius HC. Adult onset myopia- oculometric features. Acta Ophthalmologica Scand. 1995; 73: 397-401.

Franceschetti A, Gernet H. Importance of ultrasonic echography for measurements of the optical components of the eye. Tr Am Acad Ophthalmol Otol. 1965; 69: 465-73.

Franceschetti A, Luyckx J. Study of the emmetropization effect of the crystalline lens by ultrasonic echography. Am J Ophthalmol. 1966; 61: 1096-100.

Francois J, Goes F. Comparative study of ultrasonic biometry of emmetropes and myopes with special regard to the heredity of myopia. In: Gitter KA, Keeney AH, Sarin LK, Meyer D, eds. Ophthalmic Ultrasound-proceedings of the 4th international congress of ultrasonography in ophthalmology, Philadelphia. St. Louis: C.V. Mosby Co.; 1969: 165-80.

Garner LF, Yap M, Scott R. Crystalline lens power in myopia. Optom Vis Sci. 1992; 69: 863-865.

Gernet H. Oculometric findings in myopia. In: Fledelius HC, Alsbirk PH, Goldschmidt E, eds. Third International conference on myopia, Copenhagen. The Hague: Dr W. Junk Publishers. Doc Ophthalmol Proc Series. 1981; 28: 71-7.

Gilmartin B. A review of the role of sympathetic innervation of the ciliary muscle in ocular accommodation. Ophthal Physiol Opt. 1986; 6: 23-37.

Gilmartin B, Bullimore MA. Sustained near-vision augments inhibitory sympathetic innervation of the ciliary muscle. Clin Vis Sci. 1987; 1: 197-208.

Gilmartin B, Bullimore MA. Adaptation of tonic accommodation to sustained visual tasks in emmetropia and late-onset myopia. Optom Vis Sci. 1991; 68: 22-6.

Gilmartin B, Bullimore MA, Rosenfield M, Winn B. Ciliary muscle tonus and innervation in late-onset myopia. Invest Ophthalmol Vis Sci (Suppl). 1989a; 30: 325.

Gilmartin B, Bullimore MA, Rosenfield M, Winn B, Owens H. Pharmacological effects on accommodative adaptation. Optom Vis Sci. 1992; 69: 276-82.

Gilmartin B, Hogan RE. The relationship between tonic accommodation and ciliary muscle innervation. Invest Ophthalmol Vis Sci. 1985a; 26: 1024-9.

Gilmartin B, Hogan RE. The role of sympathetic nervous system in ocular accommodation and ametropia. Ophthal Physiol Opt. 1985b; 5: 91-3.

Gilmartin B, Winfield NR. The effect of topical beta-adrenoceptor antagonist on accommodation in emmetropia and myopia. Vis Res. 1995;35:1305-12.

Gilmartin B, Winn B, Pugh JR, Owens H. Ciliary muscle innervation and predisposition to late-onset myopia. Optom Vis Sci (Suppl). 1989b; 66: 217.

Gobba FM, Broglia A, Sarti R, Luberto F, Cavalleri A. Visual fatigue in VDT operators: objective measures and relation to environmental conditions. Int Arch Occup Environ Health. 1988; 60: 81-7.

Goldschmidt E. On the etiology of myopia- an epidemiological study. Acta Ophthalmol (Suppl). 1968; 98: 1-172.

Goldstein JH, Schneekloth BB. Spasm of the near reflex: a spectrum of anomalies. Surv Ophthalmol. 1996; 40: 269-78.

Goss DA. Clinical accommodation and heterophoria findings preceding juvenile onset of myopia. Optom Vis Sci. 1991; 68: 110-6.

Grosvenor TP. Myopia and its development. In: Primary Care Optometry. New York: Professional Press Books/Fairchild Publications; 1989: 57-89.

Grosvenor T, Scott R. Three-year changes in refraction and its components in youth-onset and early adult-onset myopia. Optom Vis Sci. 1993; 70: 677-83.

Gur S, Ron S. Contrast sensitivity and the near point of accommodation after work with a visual display unit. Isr J Med Sci. 1992; 28: 618-21.

Haider M, Kundi M, Weibenbock M. Worker strain related to VDUs with differently coloured characters. In: Grandjean E, Vigliani E, eds. Ergonomic Aspects of Visual Display Terminals. London: Taylor & Francis; 1980: 53-64.

Harrington S, Watanabe DS, Jiang BC, White JM. Accommodative adaptation does not alter the accommodative stimulus/response function. Optom Vis Sci (Suppl). 1992; 69: 110.

Holm E. The pathogenesis of reading myopia. Acta Ophthalmol. 1926; 3: 233-44.

Hung GK. Adaptation model of accommodation and vergence. Ophthal Physiol Opt. 1992; 12: 319-26.

Hung GK, Ciuffreda KJ, Rosenfield M. Proximal contribution to a linear static model of accommodation and vergence. Ophthal Physiol Opt. 1996; 16: 31-41.

Hung GK, Ciuffreda KJ, Semmlow JL. Static vergence and accommodation: population norms and orthoptic effects. Doc Ophthalmol. 1986; 62: 165-79.

Hung GK, Semmlow JL. Static behavior of accommodation and vergence: computer simulation of an interactive dual-feedback system. IEEE Trans Biomed Engn. 1980; BME-27: 439-47.

Jaschinski-Kruza W. Transient myopia after visual work. Ergonomics. 1984; 27: 1181-9.

Kikkawa Y, Sato T. Elastic properties of the lens. Exp Eye Res. 1963; 2: 210-5.

Kran B, Ciuffreda KJ. Non-congruent stimuli and tonic accommodation. Am J Optom Physiol Opt. 1988; 65: 703-9.

Lancaster WB, Williams ER. New light on the theory of accommodation, with practical applications. Trans Amer Acad Ophth Oto-Laryng. 1914; 19:170-95.

Lepper RD, Trier HG. Measurement of accommodative changes in human eyes by means of a high-resolution ultrasonic system. In: Ossoinig KC, ed. Ophthalmic Echography, Proceedings of the 10th SIDUO Congress. Dordrecht: Martinus Nijhoff/ Dr. W. Junk Publishers. Doc Ophthalmol Proc Series. 1987; 48: 157-62.

Liu JS, Lee M, Jang J, Ciuffreda KJ, Wong JH, Grisham D, Stark L. Objective assessment of accommodation orthoptics: dynamic insufficiency. Am J Optom Physiol Opt. 1979; 56:285-294.

Lograno MD, Reibaldi A. Receptor responses in fresh human ciliary muscle. Br J Ophthalmol. 1986; 87: 379-85.

Luckiesh M, Moss FK. Ocular changes in school children during the 5th and 6th grades. Am J Optom. 1939; 16: 443-50.

McBrien NA, Millodot M. A biometric investigation of late-onset myopic eyes. Acta Ophthalmol. 1987; 65: 461-8.

McBrien NA, Millodot M. Differences in adaptation of tonic accommodation with refractive state. Invest Ophthalmol Vis Sci 1988; 29: 460-9.

Mei Q, Rong Z. Early signs of myopia in Chinese schoolchildren. Optom Vis Sci. 1994; 71: 14-6.

Michaels D. Visual optics and refraction, 2nd ed St. Louis:Mosby;1980: 398-9.

Miwa T, Tokoro T. Accommodative hysteresis of refractive errors in light and dark fields. Optom Vis Sci. 1993; 70: 323-7.

Mordi JA. Accommodation, aging and presbyopia. PhD thesis, SUNY/State College of Optometry, New York; 1991.

Morgan MW. Stimulus to and response of accommodation. Can J Optom. 1968; 30: 71-8.

Morse SE, Smith EL III. Long-term adaptational aftereffects of accommodation are associated with distal dark focus and not with late onset myopia. Invest Ophthalmol Vis Sci (Suppl). 1993; 34: 1308.

Murch GM. Visual fatigue and operator performance with DVST and raster displays. Proc SID. 1983; 24: 53-61.

Nyman KG, Bengt GK, Voss M. Work with video display terminals among office employees. Scand J Work Environ Health. 1985; 11: 483-7.

Ong E. Oculomotor interactions and nearwork-induced transient myopia in late-onset myopes. Ph.D. Thesis, State University of New York, State College of Optometry, 1996.

Ong E, Ciuffreda KJ. Nearwork-induced transient myopia- a critical review. Doc Ophthalmol. 1995; 91: 57-85.

Ong E, Ciuffreda KJ, Rosenfield M. Accommodation, vergence and nearwork-induced transient myopia. Optom Vis Sci (Suppl). 1994; 71: 129.

Ong E, Ciuffreda KJ, Rosenfield M. Effect of target proximity on transient myopia induced by equidioptric stimuli. Optom Vis Sci. 1995; 72: 502-5.

Ong E, Ciuffreda KJ, Rosenfield M. Accommodation, vergence and transient myopia. Invest Ophthalmol Vis Sci (Suppl). 1996; 37: 164.

Ong E, Ciuffreda KJ, Tannen B. Static accommodation in congenital nystagmus. Invest Ophthalmol Vis Sci. 1993; 34: 194-204.

Ostberg O. Accommodation and visual fatigue in display work. In: Grandjean E. Vigliani E, eds. Ergonomic Aspects of Visual Display Terminals. London: Taylor & Francis; 1980: 41-52.

Owens DA. Near work, acccommodative tonus, and myopia. In: Grosvernor T, Flom M, eds. Refractive Anomalies: Research and Clinical Applications. Boston: Butterworth-Heinemann; 1991: 318-44.

Owens DA, Harris D. Oculomotor adaptation and the development of myopia. Invest Ophthalmol Vis Sci (Suppl). 1980; 80.

Owens DA, Harris D, Owens RL, Francis EL. Tonic accommodation and late-onset myopia: a longitudinal investigation. Invest Ophthalmol Vis Sci (Suppl). 1989; 30: 325.

Owens DA, Wolf-Kelly K. Near work, visual fatigue and variations of oculomotor tonus. Invest Ophthalmol Vis Sci. 1987; 28: 743-9.

Pigion RG, Miller RJ. Fatigue of accommodation: Changes in accommodation after visual work. Am J Optom Physiol Opt. 1985; 62: 853-63.

Rosenfield M, Ciuffreda KJ. Cognitive demand and transient nearwork-induced myopia. Optom Vis Sci. 1994; 71: 381-5.

Rosenfield M, Ciuffreda KJ, Hung GK. The linearity of proximally-induced accommodation and vergence. Invest Ophthalmol Vis Sci. 1991; 32: 2985-91.

Rosenfield M, Ciuffreda KJ, Hung GK, Gilmartin B. Tonic accommodation: a review. I. Basic aspects. Ophthal Physiol Opt. 1993; 13: 266-84.

Rosenfield M, Ciuffreda KJ, Hung GK, Gilmartin B. Tonic accommodation: a review. II. Accommodation adaptation and clinical aspects. Ophthal Physiol Opt. 1994b; 14: 1-13.

Rosenfield M, Ciuffreda KJ, Novogrodsky L. Contribution of accommodation and disparity-vergence to transient nearwork-induced myopic shifts. Ophthal Physiol Opt. 1992a; 12: 433-6.

Rosenfield M, Ciuffreda KJ, Novogrodsky L, Yu A, Gillard M. Sustained near-vision does indeed induce myopia! Invest Ophthalmol Vis Sci (Suppl). 1992b; 33: 710.

Rosenfield M, Gilmartin B. Accommodative adaptation induced by sustained disparity-vergence. Am J Optom Physiol Opt. 1988a; 65: 118-26.

Rosenfield M, Gilmartin B. Temporal aspects of accommodative adaptation. Optom Vis Sci. 1989; 66: 229-34.

Rosenfield M, Gilmartin B. Effect of target proximity on the open-loop accommodative response. Optom Vis Sci. 1990; 67: 74-9.

Sato T. The causes and prevention of acquired myopia. Yokohama: Helarudo Printing Co., Ltd.; 1957.

Shen CS, Chiu SB, Wang AH, Ko LS. Accommodation and visual fatigue in visual display terminal (VDT) work. Acta Ophthlamol (Suppl). 1988; 185: 175-6.

Shum PJT, Ko LS, Ng CL, Lin SL. A biometric study of ocular changes during accommodation. Am J Ophthalmol. 1993; 115: 76-81.

Soriano HM. Echographic findings in accommodation. In: Ossoinig KC, ed. Ophthalmic Echography, Proceedings of the 10th SIDUO Congress. Dordrecht: Martinus Nijhoff/Dr. W. Junk Publishers. Doc Ophthalmol Proc Series. 1987; 48: 163-9.

Stenström S. Untersuchungen über die variation und kovariation der optischen elemente des menschlichen auges. Acta Ophthalmol (Suppl). 1946; 26. Cited in Sorsby A. Biology of the eye as an optical system. In: Tasman W, ed. Duane's Clinical Ophthalmology, vol. 1. Philadelphia: J. B. Lippincott Co; 1994; chap. 34: 1-17.

Stenström S. Variations and correlations of the optical components of the eye. In: Sorsby A, ed. Modern Trends in Ophthalmology, vol. 2, 2nd ed. New York: Paul B. Hoeber, Inc.; 1947: 87-102.

Stenstrom S. Investigation of the variation and the covariation of the optical elements of human eyes. Trans Woolf D. Am J Optom Arch Am Acad Optom. 1948; 25: 218-32, 286-99, 340-50, 388-97, 438-49, 496-504.

Storey JK, Rabie EP. Ultrasound- a research tool in the study of accommodation. Ophthal Physiol Opt. 1983; 3: 315-20.

Strang NC, Winn B, Gilmartin B. Repeatability of post-task regression of accommodation in emmetropia and late-onset myopia. Ophthal Physiol Opt. 1994; 14: 88-91.

Suzuki R. Neuronal influence on the mechanical activity of the ciliary muscle. Br J Ophthalmol. 1983; 78: 591-7.

Takahashi M. Accommodative response in observing CRT display. J Sci Labour. 1983; 59: 345-53.

Tan RKT, O'Leary DJ. Accommodation characteristics before and after near work. Clin Exp Optom. 1988; 71: 165-9.

Tornqvist G. The relative importance of the parasympathetic and sympathetic nervous systems for accommdoation in monkeys. Invest Ophthalmol Vis Sci. 1967; 6: 612-7.

Tron EJ. Variationsstatistische Untersuchungen u. Refraktion. Graefes Arch Ophthalmol. 1929; 122: 1. Cited in Sorsby A, Benjamin B, Davey JB, Sheridan M, Tanner JM. Emmetropia and its aberrations, a study in the correlation of the optical components of the eye. Med Res Council Special Report Series No. 293. London: Her Majesty's Stationery Office; 1957.

Van Alphen GWHM. On emmetropia and ametropia. Ophthalmol (Suppl). 1961; 142: 1-92.

Van Alphen GWHM. The adrenergic receptors of the intraocular muscles of the human eye. Invest Ophthalmol. 1976; 15: 502-5.

Young T. On the Mechanism of the Eye. Phil Trans B. 1801; 1: 23-88.

FOOTNOTE 1

A portion of this chapter was previously published, Ong and Ciuffreda (1995).

FOOTNOTE 2

While this phenomenon has been historically referred to in the literature as nearwork-induced transient myopia, the more appropriate term should be nearwork-induced transient pseudomyopia. It is acknowledged that no actual shift in the far point of refraction occurred, but that the post-task measurements reflected the accommodative adaptation occurring under visual feedback conditions superimposed on the baseline far point of refraction. However, for simplicity and for consistency with the literature, the use of the term "nearwork-induced transient myopia" will be retained for the purpose of the present monograph.

CHAPTER 5 BIOMECHANICAL MECHANISMS IN MYOPIGENESIS

Most studies link myopia to increased axial length. Von Arlt (1856) provided some of the earliest evidence. In his dissections of myopic eyes, he found all of them to be elongated posteriorly. This was later confirmed by Donders (1864), who used ophthalmometric measurements to demonstrate that the myopia was caused by lengthening of the eye and not changes in the cornea. He found that the corneas of myopic eyes were as flat or even flatter than those of emmetropic eyes. Nearly a century later, Stenstrom (1948), and later Sorsby et al. (1961), likewise suggested that axial length was the primary determinant of refractive status. In addition, others provided further evidence for its primary role in adult myopic onset and progression (Adams 1987, McBrien and Millodot 1987, Curtin 1985, 1988, Grosvenor and Scott 1991, Adams and McBrien 1992a, Grosvenor 1994, Jiang and Woessner 1996). Thus, while the effect is clear, the mechanisms are not. From a biomechanical perspective, both accommodation and convergence have been proposed as being responsible for producing myopia, but the evidence remains sketchy. At times, it appears that there are more hypotheses than facts. In this chapter, we will provide a historical overview and critical review of the literature in this area.

ACCOMMODATION

Accommodation and Biomechanics

Support for the role of accommodation in myopigenesis in humans can be gleaned from studies using pharmacological agents. Parasympatholytics paralyze accommodation while preserving convergence. Hence, if accommodation plays a role in myopic development, then any interference with the accommodative mechanism should clearly impact on the development of myopia. The arrest of myopia should result from the chronic application of such an agent. The predicted results for binocular (Dyer 1979) and monocular atropinization (Bedrossian 1978, 1979) in young myopic children were found. Atropinization resulted in a mean reduction of myopia in the treated eyes. Conversely, the myopia in the non-atropinized eyes continued to show progression. And, when the treatment was reversed, the

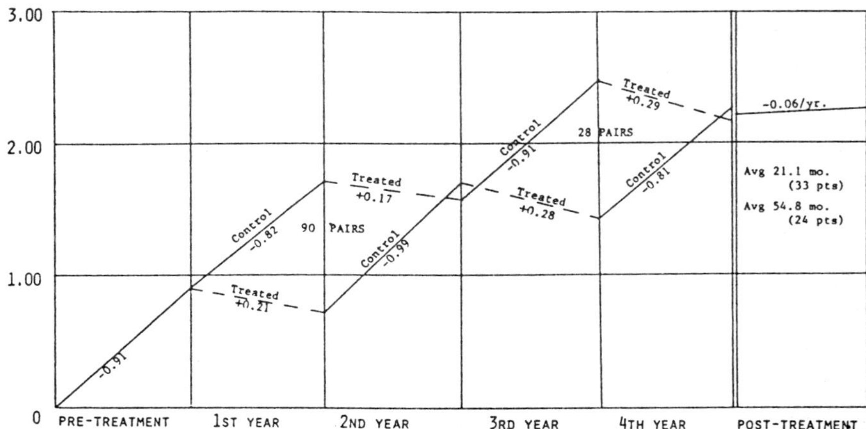

Figure 5-1 : Annualized change in refraction for all study periods (Reprinted with permission, Bedrossian 1979).

effect likewise reversed (Bedrossian 1978, 1979) (Figure 5-1). Long-term follow-up showed stabilization of refractive error in atropinized eyes. Accordingly, the results of these studies implicated the important role of the local biomechanics of accommodation in myopic progression.

The effect of parasympatholytic agents as well as other means of preventing accommodation in either visually-restricted or visually-deprived animals has also been widely documented. The administration of atropine effectively prevented myopic development. Myopia was not found in atropinized lid-sutured tree shrews (McKanna and Casagrande 1981). Moreover, Wallman et al. (1981) showed that the axial myopia induced as a result of form deprivation in chicks was reduced following ciliary nerve section, although it failed to abolish the development of myopia entirely. For primates living in enclosed environments, it was found to cause a reduction in myopia of 0.50D (Young 1965), although this effect was not consistently found across species. Similarly, only one of the two species of monkeys studied exhibited such an arrest of myopia (atropine) in a later study (Raviola and Wiesel 1980).

In contrast to these studies supporting to varying degrees the role of accommodation in the etiology of myopia, other studies in humans and lower species found counterevidence. The results of Luedde (1932), who also employed monocular cycloplegia, were diametrically opposite to that of Bedrossian (1978, 1979). Despite the monocular administration of a cycloplegic agent, myopic progression was essentially arrested in *both* eyes, thus leading him to conclude that convergence was the primary factor (see next section). By the same token, clinically reported cases of unilateral myopia would argue against both accommodation and convergence, as these oculomotor systems typically function synergistically.

Alternatively, a totally different mechanism may be responsible. Work on chicks (McBrien et al. 1993) has shown that the action of atropine on the course of myopia involved a nonaccommodative route. The administration of atropine markedly reduced the experimentally-induced myopia as well as the related biometric changes. It was proposed that the non-accommodative route involved the alteration of local retinal neurotransmitters influencing ocular growth. These neurotransmitters were believed to be regulated by atropine. See Chapter 7. In addition, Raviola and Wiesel (1985) found that removal of the ciliary ganglion, which interrupted the parasympathetic innervation to the ciliary muscles, still resulted in lid fusion myopia in rhesus monkeys. In other species, Schaeffel et al. (1990) demonstrated that optically-induced myopia and hyperopia occurred in chicks in the absence of accommodation. Moreover, despite the loss of accommodation as a consequence of lesioning of the Edinger-Westphal nucleus, myopia with correlated axial elongation still occurred with the use of a negative inducing lens versus a positive treatment lens. Similarly, Troilo et al. (1987) showed that form deprivation in chicks resulted in axial myopia despite optic nerve section. In all cases, despite the virtual elimination of the accommodative input by various means, the consistent finding of axial-based myopia suggests that some other mechanism must be responsible. *It is possible that it is not the loss of accommodation per se but rather the optical defocus and resultant image degradation occurring as a result of the absence or marked reduction of accommodation that was the triggering mechanism of the myopia* (Gwiazda et al. 1993, Held et al. 1994, Goss and Wickham 1995). See Chapters 6 and 7.

Accommodation, Intraocular Pressure and Myopia

Axial length has been reported to increase secondary to presumed stretching of the ocular coats following excessive and sustained accommodation and/or vergence, optical defocus, and the direct mechanical effects of increased intraocular pressure. Proponents of accommodation as the primary causative mechanism of myopigenesis have generally suggested an accommodatively-related increase in intraocular pressure and its related stress on the ocular coats as being responsible for this posterior pole stretch. Young (1977, 1981b) suggested that myopia appeared to develop in a two-phase process:

(1) Phase One: This consisted of excessive accommodation due to prolonged near work, which over time would lead to an inability to relax accommodation fully when attempting to focus into the distance. Accommodation would thus be maintained at a level of 0.5-1.5D rather than

0.25D or so based on the hyperfocal refraction (Rosenfield et al. 1992). This stage involved a lenticular-related change based on habitual alteration of the tonic innervation to the ciliary muscle, and it was reversible. If true, then early intervention (e.g., high plus near add, accommodative facility therapy, auditory biofeedback therapy, relaxation exercises, and/or frequent rest periods during prolonged periods of nearwork) should inhibit, prevent, or even reverse this lens-based myopic phase. However, if this pseudomyopic level were maintained for a sufficiently long period of time, it would proceed to phase two. See Chapter 4.

(2) Phase Two: Due to this prolonged overaccommodation, the smooth ciliary muscle would effectively change its habitual tonic state to reflect this new level of distant accommodation (Young 1981b). Moreover, the increased vitreous pressure associated with accommodation (but see later discussion in this chapter) (Young 1981a) would lead to a mechanical stress-induced increase in vitreous chamber length, thus producing axial-based myopia (Young 1977).

The significant role played by the ciliary muscle tone in the regulation of ocular growth was also espoused earlier by Holm (1926); also see van Alphen's ideas (1961) in Chapter 4 and later in this chapter. According to Holm's theory, prolonged and excessive nearwork resulted in increased innervation to the ciliary muscle. This augmented its tone which subsequently stimulated ocular growth and hence gave rise to axial myopia.

Another lens-based theory was developed by Coleman (1970). The most distinctive feature of Coleman's theory of accommodation was the significant role ascribed to the posterior lens and vitreous during the process of accommodation. Anatomical examination demonstrated contiguity of the lens and vitreous body via the zonules. This theory proposed that during accommodation, ciliary muscle contraction displaced the ora serrata anteriorly, therefore drawing the vitreous body against the posterior lens surface. This resulted in a relative pressure gradient between the aqueous and vitreous compartments. Vitreous chamber pressure increased, while anterior chamber pressure decreased proportionally. Sustained accommodation led to sustained and increased vitreous pressure. It was also suggested to play an important role in the development of axial myopia (Young 1975, 1981b, Bell 1980). The increased vitreous pressure exerted stress on the ocular structures as evidenced ultimately by axial elongation, thinning of the sclera in the posterior pole, and the presence of crescents and retinal stretch lesions. Applying Coleman's theory, Bell (1980) indicated that the sclera responded to the stress from the increased vitreous pressure by expansion. Upon removal of this stress, the sclera was believed to recover slowly, although failing to regain its original dimensions and thus demonstrating some partial permanent plastic deformation. However, he qualified this notion by indicating that the effect may not be universal. The primary index of whether or not a person became myopic depended largely on the scleral integrity and/or its ability to resist stress. Pressure in excess of that safely allowed by the scleral modulus of elasticity, or repeated and prolonged abnormally high pressure, could potentially lead to axial elongation.

A similar mechanism was proposed by Kelly (1981). According to him, during accommodation the ciliary body draws the vitreous body anteriorly. This applies pressure onto the zonules, thereby blocking the zonular gaps and interfering with aqueous outflow. In turn, this would lead to increased intraocular pressure causing the stress on the sclera to be elevated by a factor of ten, and ultimately leading to expansion of the globe. Thus, the mechanism of myopic development was similar to that of glaucoma, except that in the former case expansion of the globe occurred. Consequently, he referred to myopia as "juvenile expansile glaucoma." However, the Coleman theory and any vitreous-based notion is cast into serious doubt based on data from Fisher (1983), who observed normal accommodative ability in a patient who had a complete vitrectomy.

A more indirect and circuitous mechanical effect of excessive accommodation on axial length leading to the development of myopia was reported by Newman (1929). He proposed that prolonged near work was the cause of acquired myopia, with it being axial in nature and occurring during the early school years. According to Newman, with increased accommodation, tension is exerted on the elastic lamina of the choroid and as a result, the vitreous body becomes compressed. And, with excessive accommodation, the ciliary muscle is "strained" and "fatigued." Over time, such excessive accommodation would result in stretching of the elastic lamina of the choroid, thereby increasing its antero-posterior diameter. Stretching would in turn adversely affect ocular nutrition and thereby "weaken" the eye. Unable to withstand the increase in intraocular pressure, the eye would stretch further, resulting in chorioretinal degeneration and posterior staphyloma. As the axial length increased, the need for accommodation would decrease. And, finally, with less contraction of the ciliary muscle, it would atrophy. However, there are several serious problems with this theory. First, the sclera and not just the choroid must stretch to produce axial elongation. Second, staphyloma is a relatively rare occurrence in myopic eyes. And, lastly, there is no evidence for ciliary muscle atrophy in youthful myopic eyes.

Many of these accommodation theories hinge on the notion of an increase in intraocular pressure, or more specifically vitreous pressure, during increased accommodation. Therefore, it is only appropriate to review the literature on accommodation and its effect on intraocular/vitreous pressure.

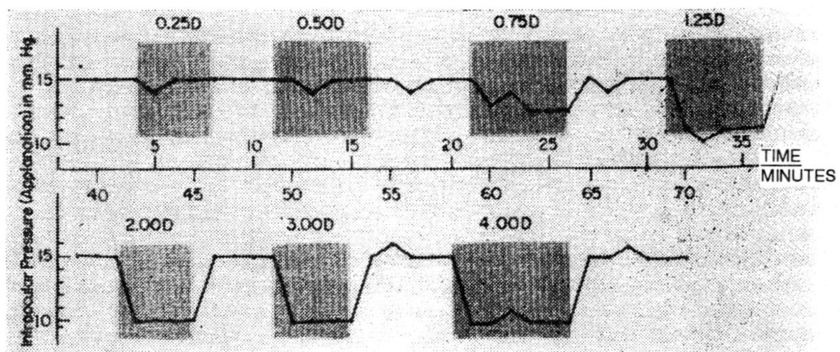

Figure 5-2 : The effect of graded accommodation on intraocular pressure. Shaded areas represent duration of accommodation, the magnitude of which is recorded in diopters above each interval. White areas represent complete relaxation. The record shows the readings at 1 minute intervals throughout the 70 minutes of the experiment. The results of the first 37 minutes appear in the upper tracing, those of the remaining minutes appear in the lower tracing (Reprinted with permission, Armaly and Rubin 1961).

Accommodation and Intraocular Pressure

As early as 1898, Hess and Heine reported that intraocular pressure did not increase with maximal contraction of the ciliary muscle. In fact, Duke-Elder (1938) even suggested that accommodation assisted in reducing intraocular pressure by causing constriction of the anterior ciliary arteries and dilation of the ciliary veins resulting in a widening of the anterior chamber angle to assist aqueous outflow. The majority of subsequent studies consistently demonstrated a decrease in intraocular pressure with increased accommodation (but see later discussion in this chapter). Tonographic studies showed higher C values, i.e., facilitated aqueous outflow, with increased accommodation, thereby resulting in a decrease in intraocular pressure.

Tonometric studies supported the above findings. A small but statistically significant reduction in intraocular pressure (1-6mm Hg) was demonstrated with increased accommodation (0-4D) (Armaly and Burian 1958, Armaly and Rubin 1961, Armaly and Jepson 1962, Mauger et al. 1984, Young and Leary 1991), with intraocular pressure decreasing in an exponential fashion. A minimum accommodative threshold of 0.50D and a saturation effect for accommodative stimuli at 1.50-2.50D or higher (Armaly and Rubin 1961) were evident (Figure 5-2), with the maximum reduction occurring primarily during the initial 30 seconds (Mauger et al. 1984). Thus, the range over which accommodation differentially reduced intraocular pressure was quite narrow, but included much of the typical near working distances. Confirmation of these alterations in intraocular pressure was reported using various pharmacological agents. For example, phenylephrine, which acts on the pupil but not the ciliary muscle, failed to produce any such effect; in contrast, cyclopentolate which is a cycloplegic, either reduced or eliminated the accommodative effect on intraocular pressure (Armaly and Rubin 1961).

To explain the finding of decreased intraocular pressure, it has been suggested that the mechanical action produced by contraction of the ciliary muscle caused the ciliary body either to pull away from the anterior chamber angle (Allen and Burian 1965) or to cause a tighter packing of the muscle bundles (Bill 1975). In the former case, it would aid in opening the trabecular meshwork, whereas in the latter case it would lead to the separation of the lamellae in the trabecular meshwork. Either mechanism would result in reduction of resistance at the meshwork level, which in turn would facilitate aqueous outflow and therefore reduce intraocular pressure in the anterior chamber.

However, in contrast to using indirect and non-invasive means of assessing intraocular pressure, Coleman and Trokel (1969) employed manometry which provided a direct measure of intraocular pressure in the aqueous chamber and found diametrically opposite results. An attempt at accommodation by the subject to an unspecified level resulted in an increase in intraocular pressure of 2-4 mm Hg. Since the study was performed on only a single subject, however, it is not possible to determine if these small changes were either significant or generalizable. Furthermore, since the subject attempted to accommodate with full cycloplegia, it is possible that facial maneuvers and squeezing of the globe by the lids during this difficult task produced the increase in intraocular pressure.

All the above studies dealt primarily with conventional intraocular pressure and hence involved measurements related to the aqueous chamber. However, the eye is composed of two basic compartments, the aqueous chamber anteriorly and the vitreous chamber posteriorly, with the latter occupying a much greater volume of the eye. Hence, the role of the vitreous in the development of myopia assumes one of greater importance, since myopic changes are characterized by increases in posterior vitreal chamber length.

Therefore, subsequent studies in animals extended the notion of increased intraocular pressure to include the vitreal chamber. For example, Suzuki's radiographic study (1973) on cats reported a transient increase in vitreous pressure with the initiation of accommodation. Other studies attempted to draw a distinction between intraocular (i.e., anterior) and vitreous chamber pressures. The existence of a relative pressure gradient within the eye was determined with the use of a differential double pressure transducer (Young 1981a). Simultaneous manometry of the anterior and posterior chambers in animals was performed, while the ciliary muscle was electrically stimulated. Results revealed a reciprocal relation between the anterior and vitreous chamber pressures, with decreased pressure in the anterior chamber occurring with a correlated increase in vitreal chamber pressure (Coleman 1970, Coleman and Young 1972). Primate studies utilizing a radiosonde type of pressure transducer also revealed the existence of this pressure gradient (Young 1975). The vitreous chamber pressure increased linearly with the accommodative demand (Young 1975). In the monkey, this increase was approximately 1 mm Hg per diopter of accommodative stimulus (Young 1975). It was maintained with sustained accommodation (Young 1981b). Young postulated that during accommodation, the ciliary muscle pulled on the choroid. The inward vector force from the choroid exerted pressure on the vitreous body, which caused the latter's pressure to increase. In addition, the choroidal pressure also increased. The continuous pressure on the choroid would lead to a reduced blood supply for both the choroid and retina, thus weakening these structures and causing them to thin and stretch. In contrast, van Alphen (1961) reported that the vitreous pressure increase generated by the choroid amounted to less than 2 mmHg. Contrary to Young's hypothesis, he believed this increase in vitreous pressure might actually *shield the sclera.* The increased choroidal tension and vitreous chamber pressure *reduced* the pressure in the suprachoroidal space, so that the increased stress from the vitreous was in fact not transmitted to the sclera (Hess and Heine 1898, van Alphen 1961).

TABLE 5-1: SUMMARY RESULTS OF INTRAOCULAR PRESSURE AS A FUNCTION OF REFRACTIVE GROUP

INVESTIGATION	INTRAOCULAR PRESSURE (mm Hg)		
	MYOPES	EMMETROPES	HYPEROPES
Edwards & Brown (1993)	13.69		11.55
Edwards, Chun & Leung (1993)	15.36	13.96	
David, Zangwill, Tessler & Yassur (1985)	14.19	14.87	15.10,16.00
Barraquer (1974)	19		10
Tomlinson & Phillips (1970)	15.49	14.74	13.91
Abdalla & Hamdi (1970)			
11-20y	15.73, 14.61	14.05	
21-30y	14.53, 14.48	13.72	
31-40y	14.70, 16.58	14.19	
41-50y	16.05, 15.33	14.39	
> 50y	16.03, 16.00	14.87	

An association between intraocular pressure and myopia has previously been noted, with myopes in general exhibiting slightly higher intraocular pressure relative to hyperopes (Abdalla and Hamdi 1970, Tomlinson and Phillips 1970, Barraquer 1974, David et al. 1985, Edwards and Brown 1993, Edwards et al. 1993) (see Table 5-1 and later discussion in this chapter). Theoretically, this difference in intraocular pressure translates into a proportional change in stress on the ocular coats, assuming all other factors remain constant (Friedman 1966). A more direct link between accommodation and mechanical stress has been suggested by Kelly (1981), who stated that this mechanical stress increased tenfold with a 50% increase in accommodation, with prolonged stress leading to expansion of the globe. However, these theoretical values seem to be grossly overstated. Careful mathematical and experimental analyses in these areas should be conducted.

The tenuous association between intraocular pressure and axial expansion was investigated in detail by van Alphen (1986). His work demonstrated an expansion of the denuded (e.g., sclera removed from ciliary body and beyond posteriorly) globe with normal intraocular pressure. His in vitro experiment demonstrated that expansion of these human eyes occurred axially as the eye was perfused with saline, which resulted in increased intraocular pressure. The maximum inflation pressure used was 14 mm Hg. Enlargement was almost exclusively found originating and expanding posteriorly from the region of the ciliary body, implicating the potentially significant role played by ciliary tonus in determining choroidal tension and the resultant net pressure on the sclera, thereby regulating the stretch of the latter. Despite the fact that the choroid did expand, which in fact is to be expected to occur due to its highly elastic balloon-like nature, this result says nothing about its effect on the sclera. In fact, were the sclera intact, clearly no such axial elongation would have occurred at the normal physiological intraocular pressures used. One must also remember that the collagenous sclera is one of the toughest materials of the human body. This was reinforced by the finding that the expansion only occurred at areas of scleral denudation. Although van Alphen (1990) subsequently showed that accommodation increased choroidal tension, nonetheless, he also indicated that accommodation did not lead to myopia. In fact, it actually appeared to prevent axial elongation by *reducing* pressure on the sclera itself as mentioned earlier (see Chapter 4 for a discussion of van Alphen's emmetropization factors).

In support of the above notion, it has been argued that the mechanical effects of accommodation are constrained by the physical strength of the ciliary muscle, which exhibits a peak force of approximately 0.5-0.6g (van Alphen 1961, Suzuki 1983, Lograno and Reibaldi 1986). In addition, it is constrained by the anatomy. Although the ciliary muscle has its origin in the scleral spur, any spread of force during its contraction would be local and thus not have impact on the posterior pole as speculated by Collicott (1996). During accommodation, the choroidal tension likewise increased by 0.6g, suggesting that all of the force from the ciliary muscle was exerted on the choroid. While this caused the vitreous chamber pressure to *increase* by less than 2 mm Hg, nonetheless, the suprachoroidal pressure *decreases* by 1mm

Hg. This suggests that the pressure on the sclera itself actually *decreases* during accommodation. Therefore, in all likelihood, the direct mechanical effects of accommodation may not assume a critical role in the elongation of the eye.

CONVERGENCE

Convergence and Biomechanics

There has been considerable theorizing but little direct evidence for the role of convergence in human myopigenesis. The convergence hypothesis implicates the mechanical action of the extraocular muscles during convergence as the basis for lengthening of the antero-posterior dimension of the eye. This included mechanical pressure on the globe itself causing increased intraocular pressure, as well as stress on the posterior globe at the extraocular muscle insertions during their contraction. Donders (1864) attributed tension of the eyes for near as the primary cause of myopia. More specifically, he enumerated the following factors as the causative mechanisms for prolongation of its axial length: (1) convergence resulting in pressure from the extraocular muscles directly on the globe, (2) passive ocular hyperemia due to the stooping position of the head during nearwork resulting in increased fluid pressure, and (3) congestion in the fundus oculi leading to softening and ectasia of the membranes, with the extension occurring primarily at the posterior pole due to the lack of support from the extraocular muscles.

Following Donder's work, von Arlt (1876) formulated his theory based on excessive convergence. He proposed that during convergence the pressure from the extraocular muscles, in particular the lateral rectus and the inferior oblique, hindered the outflow of blood from the eye. This resulted in congestion and increased intraocular pressure. Several other investigators also expressed similar opinions regarding the role of the extraocular muscles in the development of myopia. These included von Graefe (1854), Cohn (1883), Stilling (1891), and Müller (1926), although differences in opinions were apparent with respect to the particular muscles involved. The lateral and medial recti (von Graefe 1854), the superior oblique muscle (Stilling 1891), and the inferior oblique (Müller 1926) have all been incriminated as the primary offenders. In fact, Müller performed inferior oblique tenotomy in 21 patients and claimed myopic reduction as a result of this surgical procedure.

Other investigators cited more specific and direct mechanical effects of convergence as being responsible for the myopia. According to Gradle (Luedde 1932), during convergence the external recti, as a result of their anterior scleral insertion, were stretched and wrapped around part of the globe. This exerted pressure on the eye thereby causing its distention. The consequent increased axial length and ovoid shape characterizing myopic eyes in turn subjected them to even greater pressure by virtue of the increased distance between the posterior pole and the center of rotation of the eye. This led to a greater traction exerted by the external rectus during rotation. Additionally, Gradle dismissed the contribution of accommodation in the development of myopia following his evaluation of myopic progression in corrected myopes. He noted that correcting myopes with concave lenses appeared to arrest myopic progression despite the increase in accommodative demand at near following such correction. However, some clinical observations have suggested otherwise (Medina 1987a,b, Goss and Wickham 1995).

Despite the support for the role of convergence by some investigators, direct evidence is especially scarce in humans. The majority of material has consisted of anecdotal reports. In support of the convergence theory, Donders (1888) cited the case of watchmakers who generally used monocular magnifying loupes, and did not become myopic. According to Donders, the use of a monocular loupe eliminated fusional (disparity) convergence, which would in turn eliminate this potential source of pressure. However, the loupe also reduced the near accommodative demand considerably, so this has not been eliminated as a potential contributing factor.

The clinical application of monocular cycloplegia based on Donder's ideas has produced some interesting results with respect to myopia control (Luedde 1932). Presumed dissociation of the two eyes by the monocular cycloplegia resulted in arrest in the progression of myopia in all cases studied. Despite the fact that the cycloplegia was only monocularly administered, the arrest of myopia occurred binocularly. According to Luedde, sustained and excessive fusional convergence caused an increase in intraocular pressure due to compression by the extraocular muscles on the globe, with the sclera eventually yielding to the increase. However, he also acknowledged that convergence may not be the only factor. Several emmetropes and hyperopes did not become myopic. Luedde speculated that intersubject differences in ocular structure may exist. In particular, scleras with reduced resistance might be more susceptible to these external pressure effects. See later section on scleral ultrastructure in this chapter.

The work by Greene (1980) indicated that the myopic eye is classically pictured as that of a prolate spheroid, with elongation occurring predominantly in the posterior half of the globe. This implies either or both of the following: (1) the posterior half of the globe is mechanically weaker; it possesses a lower yield stress (Greene 1991), or (2) a greater concentration of forces and mechanical stresses is exerted in this area. He favored the second hypothesis. Greene contended that the extraocular muscles, in particular the obliques, exerted significant amounts of tensile stress on the posterior sclera. Moreover, he also believed that it was convergence per se that gave rise to the elevated vitreous pressure. Both of these factors imposed concentrated stress on the sclera, which in turn had the potential to cause stretch. However, once again, no evidence was presented pertaining either to the relation between convergence and intraocular pressure or the direct mechanical effects of the action of the muscles on the sclera, much less any direct evidence in support of his theories.

Convergence Stress and Strain

The theoretical mechanical aspects in axial elongation and the stress distribution on the eye were analyzed by Friedman (1966) and Greene (1980, 1991) in terms of relevant concepts in biomechanics. Stress is defined as the force per unit area, while strain refers to the deformation of a body in response to an applied force. According to Friedman (1966), the eye is subject to at least three different types of stress namely, tensile (i.e., external force acting on a body at both ends, parallel to the length, causing it to elongate), compressive (i.e, external force acting on a body to shorten it in the direction of the applied force), and shear or tangential (i.e., external force causing the movement of parallel surfaces of a solid body), which in turn are governed by the intraocular pressure, the ocular radius of curvature, and the thickness of the ocular coats. The more important tensile force is derived from a tangential component and acts circumferentially, with this force resulting in an increase in globe radius and thinning of the wall; the compressive force acts directly and centrifugally, while the shearing forces parallel to the surface are due to the difference in the physical structure of the various layers of the ocular coats. The stress imposed on the ocular shell by the vitreous pressure renders the eye under biaxial stress, i.e., being pulled equally in every direction in the plane of the ocular coat (Greene 1980, 1991). Using schematic eye values, the hypothetically-derived stress value was equivalent to 1.2 g/mm^2.

Also, based on Greene's equations, the greater the intraocular pressure, the greater the radius of curvature or the flatter the surface; furthermore, the thinner the ocular coats, the greater is the stress. Thus, the myopic eye is at a mechanical disadvantage. As mentioned earlier, slightly higher mean intraocular pressures have been found in myopic eyes (Table 5-1). In addition, increased axial lengths and flatter curvatures have also been observed (Stenstrom 1948, van Alphen 1961). And, as calculated by Friedman (1966), there is approximately a 4% stress difference for every 2.50D of axial ametropia, with this difference increasing to as much as 60% between hyperopes and myopes in extreme refractive cases. Finally, a considerably thinner choroid and retina in myopes were revealed in cross-sectional measurements of the ocular coats (Mawas 1934). Mean values obtained were 0.8 mm for normals and 0.25 mm for high myopes. This variation in thickness alone yields a difference in stress by a factor of three for myopic eyes. All of these factors combined clearly demonstrate that the myopic eye is subjected to a comparatively greater amount of stress than the eyes of other refractive groups. Friedman suggested that if the forces exerted upon the sclera were of an excessive magnitude, it would result in expansion of the globe. Moreover, he also emphasized the importance of time-dependent cumulative effects.

The eye in axial myopia is typified by distortion of the posterior region, while the anterior region remains unchanged. Greene (1991) posed specific suggestions as to why only the posterior half was affected. He indicated that the oblique muscle insertions were located in the posterior region of the eye. Analysis of the stress distribution was performed to simulate the forces imposed on the sclera when the extraocular muscles pulled tangentially against it. More specifically, the distribution of tensile and compressive stresses from the pull of the oblique muscles was calculated. Extant literature indicate that muscle attachment widths varied from 5 to 14 mm (Hogan et al. 1971), while the range of forces from oblique muscles was from 10 to 40g. Assuming a scleral thickness of 1 mm, the mechanical stress imposed by the contraction of a single oblique muscle can range from approximately 0.4g (for a 14 mm attachment width and a 10 g muscle force) to 4 g (for a 5mm attachment width and a 40g muscle force). Thus, the actual forces exerted on the globe were not equal to the forces developed by the extraocular muscle (up to 150g) and in fact were more similar to that found for maximal accommodation (~0.5g). The magnitude of this calculated stress value is increased by a factor of two when both oblique muscles pull simultaneously in opposite directions. Thinner scleral coats would clearly lead to increased stress values. The resultant compressive and tensile forces would be distributed in the plane of the sclera, with their effects being greatest at the point of application. However, one would have to measure scleral thickness in pre-myopes and find it to be thinner than in emmetropes for this notion to have relevance with respect to myopic onset; however, it may relate to myopic progression.

The stress experienced by the posterior sclera is the resultant linear summation of the stresses induced by both of the aforementioned factors, i.e., the intraocular pressure and the oblique muscles. The worst case scenario is attained for larger eyes, greater transmural pressure, narrow muscle attachment lines, higher muscle tension, thinner sclera, and close attachment between the two oblique muscles. Finally, the region between the two muscle attachments is under considerable tensile stress which is diffused laterally. In the case of the globe, the optic nerve encounters a substantial amount of tensile stress. Greene (1980, 1991) noted that at the edge of the entrance of the optic nerve into the posterior pole of the eye, the mechanical stress was augmented by a factor of 3. Such a concentration of stress effectively weakens the sclera in that region. This appears to be consistent with the occurrence of posterior staphyloma in pathologic myopia.

In addition, Greene compared the mechanical strengths of the ciliary muscle and the extraocular muscles and indicated that the mechanical effects of accommodation and convergence were limited by their corresponding sets of muscles. According to him, by virtue of the greater potential peak force capability of the medial rectus muscle (150 g) (Robinson 1964) as opposed to that exerted by the ciliary muscle (0.5-0.6 g) (van Alphen 1961, Suzuki 1983, Lograno and Reibaldi 1986), it is obvious that the mechanical action of convergence maximally overrides that of accommodation by a factor of approximately 300.

How this stress, as calculated above, theoretically translates into actual strain may be gleaned from other studies. At the same time, it may also shed light on the mechanical characteristics of the sclera. In vitro experimental studies by Greene and McMahon (1979) evaluated the factors causing scleral creep, with creep being defined as the continued increase in tissue length when exposed to a constant tensile force (Norton and Rada 1995). When the intraocular pressure in excised rabbit eyes was systematically varied, results showed that permanent scleral creep occurred when the stress was present for a substantial length of time, (Greene and McMahon 1979). However, it was only observed in young rabbit eyes and progressing at a slow rate (0.04% to 15%/hour equivalent to 0.015 to 5.63D/hour for intraocular pressures of 15 to 100 mmHg). Factors such as pressure and temperature affected the creep rate. At abnormal physiological conditions, a 1% plastic strain of the posterior sclera was evident only after 7 hours of being subjected to a pressure of 30 mm Hg (e.g., twice the normal level) at a temperature of 37^{0}C, although a creep rate of 0.06%/hour or 0.5D/day was observed under physiological conditions, i.e., 37°C and 15 mm Hg. Greene (1978) indicated that intraocular pressure was directly related to mechanical stress in rabbits, and that intraocular pressure may be a critical variable in the ultimate geometry of ocular coats.

Nonetheless, and most importantly, *no such creep was reported for adult human specimens* (Greene and McMahon 1979). However, it would be informative to repeat this work using tissue from infants and children, especially either those at risk for myopia or having just developed their myopia. Curtin (1969) also failed to demonstrate permanent deformation on human scleral strips even for forces equivalent to intraocular pressure of 100 mmHg, although some samples did exhibit permanent deformation of

1% strain following repeated cycles of stress corresponding to 100 mmHg. Of course, such intraocular pressure values are extreme and well beyond the normal physiological range.

Ku and Greene (1981) also suggested that cyclic stress could lead to environmentally-induced myopia. Transient high intraocular pressure pulses are possibly encountered in our daily lives. High pressures (110 mm Hg) have been recorded in humans by hard squinting (Coleman and Trokel 1969). Yet, in above cases, there was no evidence of axial elongation or global distortion. Thus, the human sclera is quite resistant to such forces.

Uniaxial stress-strain experiments on scleral and choroidal strips of enucleated human eyes have revealed the exponential stress-strain characteristics of the sclera, while choroidal strips demonstrated power law behavior (Graebel and van Alphen 1977). Hence, for an equivalent amount of strain, the sclera exhibited 10 times more stress than the choroid, and therefore was ten times more resistant to such pressures than the choroid. The modulus of elasticity of the anterior sclera was found to be greater than the posterior sclera (Friberg and Lace 1988).

Correlational studies (Perkins 1981a) also failed to provide strong support for the role of mechanical stress on the human sclera with respect to the enlargement of the eyeball and myopic development. Scleral stress was calculated for different individuals. Perkins determined these variables empirically using a clinical population. The subjects were divided according to the severity of the ophthalmoscopic findings, as well as their age. The normal group exhibited an absence of myopic changes, grade 1 eyes exhibited myopic crescents, and grade 2 eyes were characterized by degenerative retinal changes. The degree of myopia and axial length were directly related to the severity of fundus changes. The calculated value of scleral stress was not significantly correlated with the degree of myopia. Significant differences were only found between normal and grade 2 eyes in the oldest age group. No significant correlation was found between refractive error and scleral thickness. This lack of correlation was addressed by Perkins. He acknowledged the possibility that the use of the light scatter technique to determine scleral thickness may prove to be unreliable in the living eye, and that this may have in turn affected the calculated scleral stress results. Data were then recalculated following the replacement of the empirically-derived measures of scleral thickness with mean values obtained from measurements of enucleated eyes. A small albeit significant correlation (r =0.196) now became evident between degree of myopia and scleral stress. In addition, Perkins indicated that a better correlation might be obtained if scleral thickness were determined at the posterior pole rather than 12mm from the limbus as was performed in his study. Furthermore, their equation assumed a spherical eyeball. Since the eyeball is not a sphere, the equation might not have provided accurate results. But most importantly, the relatively low correlation obtained after the correction factor was used suggested that other factors were involved in the relation between scleral stress and axial elongation.

Convergence and Intraocular Pressure

To investigate the validity of the convergence hypothesis, one must first establish a relation between the action of the extraocular muscles and intraocular pressure. As early as 1930, eminent investigators such as Duke-Elder reported increases in intraocular pressure in dogs upon simultaneous stimulation of all of the extraocular muscles with acetylcholine (Duke-Elder 1938). Later, additional animal studies were conducted. Macri and Grimes (1957) tested adult cats. Simultaneous recording showed that succinylcholine, which caused co-contraction of all of the extraocular muscles, produced parallel changes in muscles tension and intraocular pressure in the contralateral eye (Figure 5-3). In addition, they found that increased drug dosage resulted in proportional elevations in intraocular pressure in the anterior chamber. Further proof was provided by sectioning of the extraocular muscles which reduced the intraocular pressure effect dramatically. Moreover, no increase in intraocular pressure was found when changes in muscle tension were prevented by the administration of d-tubocurarine, which paralyzed the extraocular muscles (as well as other muscles of the body). Collins et al. (1967) also found similar results. It was concluded that such vigorous, simultaneous ocular muscle contraction led to a rise in intraocular pressure. It was estimated that compression and distortion of the globe from cocontraction contributed to approximately 30% of the rise in

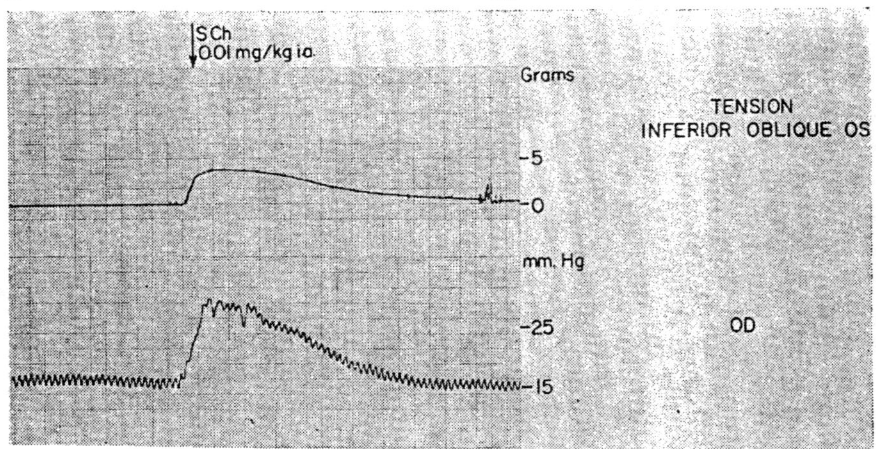

Figure 5-3 : Effect of succinylcholine on intraocular pressure and the contralateral inferior oblique muscle tension. Intraocular pressure increases synchronously with an increase of the muscle tension (Reprinted with permission, Macri and Grimes 1957).

intraocular pressure, while the remaining 70% was due to the direct and local mechanical effects of the extraocular muscles on the sclera.

The same pharmacological agent applied to human subjects (n =75) resulted in similar findings (Lincoff et al. 1955). Following administration of succinylcholine, intraocular pressure as measured with the Schiotz tonometer showed a mean rise of approximately 8 mm Hg. Sectioning of the extraocular muscles in 3 subjects (during routine extraocular muscle surgery) markedly reduced these intraocular pressure changes. Thus, the increase in intraocular pressure was secondary to simultaneous contraction of the muscles and their resultant powerful forces against the sclera.

However, the effects derived from the application of succinylcholine and other similarly acting pharmacological agents should be interpreted with considerable caution. Cocontracture *is not* equivalent to convergence. The latter is characterized by reciprocal innervation, i.e., the medial rectus of each eye is stimulated while the lateral recti are inhibited (Ciuffreda and Tannen 1995) with relatively small forces exerted, as opposed to the much more vigorous and forceful simultaneous innervation to *all* twelve extraocular muscles during cocontracture. Since succinylcholine causes the simultaneous contraction of all of the extraocular muscles, such action may result in considerable compression and traction of the whole eyeball. In fact, Collins et al. (1967) indicated that cocontracture of the muscles resulted in enophthalmos. The strong forces on the eyeball resulted in unnaturally increased compression and inward movement on the globe. Therefore this clearly *is not* an accurate representation of the action of the extraocular muscles during convergence in one's normal daily near visual activities.

More recently, intraocular pressure in 20 human subjects was evaluated with respect to the angle of horizontal gaze (Kumata et al. 1994). Intraocular pressure measurements were recorded in primary gaze as well as 15, 25 and 35 degrees to the left and right. A small but significant increase in intraocular pressure was obtained in 5 of the 6 eccentric gaze positions. The intraocular pressure increased linearly with increased deviation from the primary gaze. At the extreme left and right gaze positions of 35 degrees, the correspondingly largest increases in intraocular pressure of approximately 2.7 mm Hg and 2.1 mm Hg were reported. Similar but larger increases in intraocular pressure were found by Coleman and Trokel (1969), Saunders et al. (1981), and Moses et al. (1982). While these results do suggest extraocular muscle-induced intraocular pressure increases, sustained gaze of such extreme values is rare. Furthermore, the resultant intraocular pressure changes are within the limits of normal diurnal variation (Duke-Elder 1952, Drance 1960, Phelps et al. 1974).

If intraocular pressure is indeed a critical factor in myopigenic axial elongation, then the intraocular pressure of myopes, or perhaps more importantly either those "at risk" of becoming myopic or who are just becoming myopic, should demonstrate such an increase. Tomlinson and Phillips (1970) compared intraocular pressure as a function of refractive group using applanation tonometry. Myopes were found to exhibit significantly greater levels of intraocular pressure than hyperopes, with both groups being similar to emmetropes (Table 5-1). Furthermore, they hypothesized that myopia developed as a consequence of elevated intraocular pressure resulting from an increased level of aqueous production coupled with a reduced aqueous outflow facility. This led to distention of the eyeball. Alternatively, it was also stated that due to the inherited nature of myopic axial elongation, the resistance to aqueous outflow is greater, perhaps resulting from a flattening of the meshwork. Likewise, Abdalla and Hamdi (1970), Barraquer (1974), David et al. (1985) and Edwards and Brown (1993) found similar results, with intraocular pressures being greater in myopes, although in the former study, this trend was not reported to be evident for all age groups.

However, this difference in intraocular pressure may not directly relate to refractive status but rather to eye size. Since myopes are characterized by elongated eyes, then intraocular pressure may predictably be greater. In fact, Tomlinson and Phillips (1970) demonstrated that intraocular pressure was found to be significantly correlated with axial length ($r = +0.37$), so that eyes with greater axial lengths exhibited higher levels of intraocular pressure. This was confirmed in a subsequent study of 13 anisometropes (Tomlinson and Phillips 1972). It was reported that the longer eye of an individual had a small but significantly increased intraocular pressure (15 versus 14.15mm Hg). Partial correlation coefficients would have to be determined to segregate the factors of refractive status from eye size.

Although the above results were biased towards an increase in intraocular pressure in myopes, nonetheless, the mean difference in intraocular pressure between groups did not exceed 2 mm Hg in any study except one. This small difference is again within the normal diurnal variation of intraocular pressure in the human eye (Duke-Elder 1952, Drance 1960, Phelps et al. 1974) and simple lid closure (Coleman and Trokel 1969). Intuitively, it seems questionable how this small difference could have such a relatively large differential effect on scleral creep. The same question arises when we consider the previously discussed study on eye position (Kumata et al. 1994), which showed that the mean increase in intraocular pressure under extreme gaze positions was approximately 2-3 mm Hg. Firstly, although scleral creep was found in several studies, they used substantially higher pressures that were well outside the normal physiological range, generally exceeding 100 mm Hg. Secondly, the near reading distance is typically 40 cm. This would demand 15 or so prism diopters (8.5 degrees) of convergence for accurate bifixation and fusion. Assuming reasonable linearity in the relation between gaze position and intraocular pressure, such an angle of gaze would induce less than 0.5 mm Hg rise in intraocular pressure. In small children with considerably shorter working distances and therefore increased convergence demands, this would probably not exceed 1 mm Hg. It is inconceivable how increases in pressure of such small magnitude could have any major impact on the tough fibrous scleral tissue causing it to strain. It would be helpful to investigate the properties of the sclera and how mechanical stress affects it, especially in young eyes and in particular children "at risk" of developing myopia. In fact, a recent longitudinal study by Edwards and Brown (1996) reported that the increase in intraocular pressure typically found in myopes occurred *following* the onset of myopia. Thus, a high intraocular pressure *cannot be* the causative factor in myopigenesis.

SCLERAL ULTRASTRUCTURE

It is possible that strain characteristics may relate to differences in scleral rigidity and its ultrastructural properties. Castrén and Pohjola (1961) determined human scleral rigidity as a function of refractive group by applying Friedenwald's nomogram to measures derived from applanation and indentation tonometric techniques. Scleral rigidity for myopes was found to be significantly less than in hyperopes or emmetropes, while it was similar for the latter two groups. The corresponding scleral rigidity coefficients for myopes, hyperopes, and emmetropes were 0.0162, 0.0189, and 0.0184, respectively. However, it was later reported that the low coefficient in myopes was not due to any structural abnormalities or distensibility of the sclera, but rather to the increased eye size in myopes (Perkins 1981b). Perkins demonstrated a significant negative correlation between intraocular volume and ocular rigidity in enucleated human eyes, with smaller eyes possessing enhanced rigidity. In addition, when the subjects were divided into subgroups on the basis of age (10-40 years), the lowest scleral rigidity coefficient was found for the 15-year-old age group. This was particularly evident for the myopic group. It was thus proposed that the low ocular rigidity at 15 years of age may be a factor in myopia development, although ocular growth is nearly completed by this age (Sorsby et al. 1961, Sorsby and Leary 1970); however, late-onset myopia can still occur in some individuals, and perhaps this is a factor in its development.

Other studies have also found architectural differences of the sclera in myopes. Curtin et al. (1979) compared electron microscopic findings of the posterior sclera of normal and staphylomatous myopic eyes. These myopic scleras were characterized by a number of structural changes. This included severe thinning, narrowing and dissociation of the collagen fiber bundles, increase in extensibility, a predominantly lamellar collagen architecture, reduced fibril diameter, greater range of fibril diameters, increased prevalence of stellate fibrils, a preponderance of fibril groups with extremely fine diameters (Curtin and Teng 1958, Curtin et al. 1979) and reduced collagen content (Avetisov et al. 1984). See Chapter 7. Moreover, many of these ultrastructural scleral changes were not limited to the posterior sclera, but it was generalized and evident in the equatorial region as well (Liu et al. 1986). However, since these changes were observed in eyes that were already myopic, it was not clear from these studies whether the morphological differences were a cause or a consequence of the myopic development. More recent work on form deprived tree shrews may shed light in this area. Structural (Phillips and McBrien 1995) as well as biochemical (Norton and Rada 1995) scleral changes were reported in form deprived myopic eyes. It was thus suggested that any differences in scleral thickness or structure, albeit small, will cause the sclera to respond differently to similar amounts of stress (Phillips and McBrien 1995) and any biochemical changes have the potential for the sclera to be more distensible thus resulting in axial myopia (Norton and Rada 1995).

SUMMARY

The findings of this chapter bring out several important points. First, myopia is not primarily due to the biomechanical aspects of accommodation, vergence, and their intraocular pressure interrelationships. Furthermore, and perhaps most importantly, these small increases in intraocular pressure were found *after* and not before myopic onset. Finally, the sclera appears to be quite resistant to a variety of internally and externally based forces.

REFERENCES

Abdalla MI, Hamdi M. Applanation ocular tension in myopia and emmetropia. Br J Ophthalmol. 1970; 54: 122-5.

Adams AJ. Axial length elongation, not corneal curvature, as a basis of adult-onset myopia. Am J Optom Physiol Opt. 1987; 64: 150-2.

Adams DW, McBrien NA. A longitudinal study of adult-onset myopia and adult progression of myopia- two year refractive error and axial dimension results. Invest Ophthalmol Vis Sci (Suppl). 1992a; 33: 712.

Allen L, Burian HM. The valve action of the trabecular meshwork. Am J Ophthalmol. 1965; 59: 382-9.

Armaly MF, Burian HM. Changes in the tonogram during accommodation. Arch Ophthalmol. 1958; 60: 60-9.

Armaly MF, Jepson NC. Accommodation and the dynamics of the steady-state intraocular pressure. Invest Ophthalmol. 1962; 1: 480-3.

Armaly MF, Rubin ML. Accommodation and applanation tonometry. Arch Ophthalmol. 1961; 65: 415-23.

Avetisov ES, Savitskaya NF, Vinetskaya MI, Iomdina EN. A study of biochemical and biomechanical qualities of normal and myopic eye sclera in humans of different age groups. Metabolic Ped Systemic Ophthalmol. 1984; 7: 183-8.

Barraquer J. Coloquio sobre miopia; 1974. Cited in Kelly TSB. In: Fledelius HC, Alsbirk PH, Goldschmidt E, eds. Third International Conference on Myopia, Copenhagen. The Hague: Dr W. Junk Publishers. Doc Ophthal Proc Series. 1981; 23: 109-16.

Bedrossian RH. The effect of atropine on myopia. In: Sato T, Yamaji R, eds. Proc of the Second International Conference on Myopia. Yokohama; 1978: 81-6.

Bedrossian RH. The effect of atropine on myopia. Ophthalmol. 1979; 86: 713-7.

Bell GR. The Coleman theory of accommodation and its relevance to myopia. J Am Optom Assoc. 1980; 51: 582-8.

Bill A. Blood circulation and fluid dynamics in the eye. Physiol Rev. 1975; 55: 383-417.

Castrén JA, Pohjola S. Refraction and scleral rigidity. Acta Ophthalmol. 1961; 39: 1011-4.

Ciuffreda KJ, Tannen B. Eye Movement Basics for the Clinician. St. Louis: C.V. Mosby; 1995.

Cohn H. Hygiene of the eye in schools. Turnbull WP, ed. London: Simpkin, Marshall and Co.; 1883.

Coleman DJ. Unified model for the accommodative mechanism. Am J Ophthalmol. 1970; 69: 1063-79.

Coleman DJ, Trokel S. Direct recorded intraocular pressure variations in a human subject. Arch Ophthalmol. 1969; 82: 637-40.

Coleman DJ, Young FA. Measurement of vitreous-aqueous pressure gradient during ciliary muscle stimulation. Invest Ophthalmol Vis Sci (Suppl). 1972.

Collicott T. Emmetropia: a refractive anomaly? Optom Today. 1996; 36: 35-9.

Collins CC, Bach-y-Rita P, Loeb DR. Intraocular tension variation with oculorotary muscle tension. Am J Physiol. 1967; 213: 1039-403.

Curtin BJ. Physiopathologic aspects of scleral stress-strain. Trans Amer Ophthalmol Soc. 1969; 67: 417-61.

Curtin BJ. The Myopias: Basic Science and Clinical Management. Philadelphia: Harper & Row; 1985.

Curtin BJ. Adult myopia. Acta Ophthalmol (Suppl). 1988; 185: 78-9.

Curtin BJ, Iwamoto T, Renaldo DP. Normal and staphylomatous sclera of high myopia-an electron microscopic study. Arch Ophthalmol. 1979; 97: 912-5.

Curtin BJ, Teng CC. Scleral changes in pathological myopia. Trans Am Acad Ophthalmol Otolaryngol. 1958; 62: 777-88.

David R, Zangwill LM, Tessler Z, Yassur Y. The correlation between intraocular pressure and refractive status. Arch Ophthalmol. 1985; 103: 1812-5.

Donders FC. On the Anomalies of Accommodation and Refraction of the Eye. Trans. Moore WD. London: The New Sydenham Society; 1864.

Donders FC. Die anomalien der refraktion und akkommodation des auges. Zweiter abdruck der unter mitwirkung des verfassers von Prof. Dr. Becker herausgegebenen deutschen originalausgabe. Wien: Wilhelm Braunmueller; 1888: 350. Cited in Luedde WH. Monocular cycloplegia for the control of myopia. Am J Ophthalmol. 1932; 15: 603-10.

Drance SM. The significance of the diurnal tension variations in normal and glaucomatous eyes. Arch Ophthalmol. 1960; 64: 494-501.

Duke-Elder S. Textbook of Ophthalmology, vol. 1. St. Louis: C.V. Mosby Co.; 1938: 492-534.

Duke-Elder S. The phasic variations in the ocular tension in primary glaucoma. Am J Ophthalmol. 1952; 35: 1-21.

Dyer JA. Role of cycloplegics in progressive myopia. Ophthalmol. 1979: 86: 692-4.

Edwards MH, Brown B. Intraocular pressure in a selected sample of myopic and non-myopic Chinese children. Optom Vis Sci. 1993; 70: 15-7.

Edwards MH, Brown B. IOP in myopic children: the relationship between increases in IOP and the development of myopia. Ophthal Physiol Opt. 1996; 243-6.

Edwards MH, Chun CY, Leung SSF. Intraocular pressure in an unselected sample of 6- to 7-year-old Chinese children. Optom Vis Sci. 1993; 70: 198-200.

Fisher RF. Is the vitreous necessary for accommodation in man? Br J Ophthalmol. 1983; 67: 206.

Friberg TR, Lace JW. A comparison of the elastic properties of human choroid and sclera. Exp Eye Res. 1988; 47: 429-36.

Friedman B. Stress upon the ocular coats: Effects of scleral curvature, scleral thickness, and intra-ocular pressure. The Eye, Ear, Nose and Throat Monthly. 1966; 45: 59-66.

Goss DA, Wickham MG. Retinal-image mediated ocular growth as a mechanism for juvenile onset myopia and for emmetropization. Doc Ophthalmol. 1995; 90: 341-75.

Graebel WP, van Alphen GWHM. The elasticity of sclera and choroid of the human eye, its implications on scleral rigidity and accommodation. J Biomech Eng. 1977; 99: 203-8.

Greene PR. Mechanical aspects of myopia (PhD thesis); Cambridge: Harvard; 1978. Cited in Greene PR. Axial myopia: plastic deformation of the sclera? In: Sato T, Yamaji R, eds. Proc of the Second International Conference on Myopia. Yokohama; 1978: 81-6.

Greene PR. Mechanical considerations in myopia: relative effects of accommodation, convergence, intraocular pressure, and the extraocular muscles. Am J Optom Physiol Opt. 1980; 57: 902-14.

Greene PR. Mechanical considerations in myopia. In: Grosvenor T, Flom MC, eds. Refractive Anomalies- Research and Clinical Applications. Boston: Butterworth-Heinemann; 1991: 287-300.

Greene PR, McMahon TA. Scleral creep versus temperature and pressure in vitro. Exp Eye Res. 1979; 29: 527-37.

Grosvenor T. Refractive component changes in adult-onset myopia: evidence from five studies. Clin Exp Optom 1994; 77: 196-205.

Grosvenor T, Scott R. Comparison of refracting components in youth-onset and early adult-onset myopia. Optom Vis Sci. 1991; 68: 204-9.

Gwiazda J, Thorn F, Bauer J, Held R. Myopic children show insufficient accommodative response to blur. Invest Ophthalmol Vis Sci. 1993; 34: 690-4.

Held R, Gwiazda JE, Thorn F, Bauer JA. Changes in accommodative responsiveness are linked to the development of myopia in children. Invest Ophthalmol Vis Sci (Suppl). 1994;35:1735.

Hess C, Heine L. Arbeiten aus dem gebiete der akkommodations- lehre. Arch f Ophth. 1898; 46: 243-76. Cited in Stansbury FC. Pathogenesis of myopia-a new classification. Arch Ophthalmol. 1948; 39: 273-99.

Hogan MJ, Alvarado JA, Weddell JE. Histology of the Human Eye. Philadelphia: WB Saunders Co., 1971.

Holm E. The pathogenesis of reading myopia. Acta Ophthalmol. 1926; 3: 233-44.

Jiang BC, Woessner WM. Vitreous chamber elongation is responsible for myopia development in a young adult. Optom Vis Sci. 1996; 73: 231-4.

Kelly TSB. Myopia or expansion glaucoma. In: Fledelius HC, Alsbirk PH, Goldschmidt E, eds. Third International Conference on Myopia, Copenhagen. The Hague: Dr W. Hunk Publishers. Doc Ophthalmol Proc Series. 1981; 28: 109-16.

Ku DN, Greene PR. Scleral creep in vitro resulting from cyclic pressure pulses: applications to myopia. Am J Optom Physiol Opt. 1981; 58: 528-35.

Kumata W, Nishimoto JH, Lai C, DeLand PN. A comparison of intraocular pressure measurement in varying lateral and medial gazes. Optom Vis Sci (Suppl). 1994; 71: 106.

Lincoff HA, Ellis CH, Gerard deVoe A, deBeer EJ, Impastato DJ, Berg S, Orkin L, Magda H. The effect of succinylcholine on intraocular pressure. Am J Ophthalmol. 1955; 40: 501-10.

Liu KR, Chen MS, Ko LS. Electron microscopic studies of the scleral collagen fiber in excessively high myopia. J Formosan Med Assoc. 1986; 85: 1032-8.

Lograno MD, Reibaldi A. Receptor responses in fresh human ciliary muscle. Br J Ophthalmol. 1986; 87: 379-85.

Luedde WH. Monocular cycloplegia for the control of myopia. Am J Ophthalmol. 1932; 15: 603-10.

Macri FJ, Grimes PA. The effects of succinylcholine on the extraocular striate muscles and on the intraocular pressure. Am J Ophthalmol. 1957; 44: 221-30.

Mauger RR, Likens CP, Applebaum M. Effects of accommodation and repeated applanation tonometry on intraocular pressure. Am J Optom Physiol Opt. 1984; 61: 28-30.

Mawas J. Introduction a l'etude de la myopie et des chorioretinites myopiques. Bull Soc d'Opht de Paris 1934; 1: 549-601. Cited in Friedman B. Stress upon the ocular coats: Effects of scleral curvature, scleral thickness, and intra-ocular pressure. The Eye, Ear, Nose and Throat Monthly. 1966; 45: 59-66.

McBrien NA, Millodot M. A biometric investigation of late-onset myopic eyes. Acta Ophthalmol. 1987; 65: 461-8.

McBrien NA, Moghaddam HO, Reeder AP. Atropine reduces experimental myopia and eye enlargement via a nonaccommodative mechanism. Invest Ophthalmol Vis Sci. 1993; 34: 205-15.

McKanna JA, Casagrande VA. Atropine affects lid-suture myopia development. In: Fledelius HC, Alsbirk PH, Goldschmidt E, eds. Third International Conference on Myopia, Copenhagen. The Hague: Dr W. Junk Publishers. Doc Ophthalmol Proc Ser. 1981; 28: 187-92.

Medina A. A model for emmetropization-predicting the progression of ametropia. Ophthalmol. 1987a; 194: 133-9.

Medina A. A model for emmetropization- the effect of corrective lenses. Acta Ophthalmol. 1987b; 65: 565-71.

Moses RA, Lurie P, Wette R. Horizontal gaze position effect on intraocular pressure. Invest Ophthalmol Vis Sci. 1982;22:551-3.

Müller L. Ueber pathogenese und behandlung der kurzsichtigkeit und ihre folgen. Wien Klin Wchnsche; 1926: 39: 321-5. Cited in Stansbury FC. Pathogenesis of myopia-a new classification. Arch Ophthalmol. 1948; 39: 273-99.

Newman FA. Acquired axial myopia. Am J Ophthalmol. 1929; 12: 714-9.

Norton TT, Rada JA. Reduced extracellular matrix in mammalian sclera with induced myopia. Vis Res. 1995; 35: 1271-81.

Perkins ES. Myopia and sclera stress. In: Fledelius HC, Alsbirk PH, Goldschmidt E, eds. Third International Conference on Myopia, Copenhagen. The Hague: Dr W. Junk Publishers. Doc Ophthalmol Proc Ser. 1981a; 28: 121-7.

Perkins ES. Ocular volume and ocular rigidity. Exp Eye Res. 1981b; 33: 141-5.

Phelps CD, Woolson RF, Kolker AE, Becker B. Diurnal variation in intraocular pressure. Am J Ophthalmol. 1974; 77: 367-7.

Phillips JR, McBrien NA. Form deprivation myopia: elastic properties of sclera. Ophthal Physiol Opt. 1995; 15: 357-62.

Pruett RC. Progressive myopia and intraocular pressure: what is the linkage? a literature review. Acta Ophthalmol (Suppl). 1988; 117-27.
Raviola E, Wiesel TN. Effects of atropine on experimental myopia in macaque monkeys. Invest Ophthalmol Vis Sci (Suppl). 1980; 170-1.
Raviola E, Wiesel TN. An animal model of myopia. New Engl J Med. 1985; 312: 1609-15.
Robinson DA. The mechanics of human saccadic eye movement. J Physiol. 1964; 174: 245-64.
Rosenfield M, Ciuffreda KJ, Novogrodsky L, Yu A, Gillard M. Sustained near vision does indeed induce myopia! Invest Ophthalmol Vis Sci (Suppl). 1992; 33: 710.
Rosenfield M, Ciuffreda KJ, Rosen J. Accommodative response during distance optometric test procedures. J Am Optom Asson. 1992; 63: 614-8.
Saunders RA, Helveston EM, Ellis FD. Differential intraocular pressure in strabismus diagnosis. Ophthalmol. 1981;88:59-70.
Schaeffel F, Troilo D, Wallman J, Howland HC. Developing eyes that lack accommodation grow to compensate for imposed defocus. Vis Neurosci. 1990; 4: 177-83.
Sorsby A, Benjamin B, Sheridan M. Refraction and its components during the growth of the eye from the age of three. Med Res Council Special Report Series No. 301. London: Her Majesty's Stationery Office; 1961.
Sorsby A, Leary GA. A longitudinal study of refraction and its components during growth. Med Res Council Special Report Series no. 309. London: Her Majesty's Stationery Office; 1970.
Stenström S. Investigation of the variation and the correlation of the optical elements of human eyes, trans. Woolf D. Am J Optom Arch Am Acad Optom. 1948; 25: 218-32, 286-99, 340-50, 388-97, 438-49, 496-504.
Stilling J. Ueber das wachsthum der orbita und dessen beziehungen zur refraction. Arch f Augenh; 1891: 22: 47-60. Cited in Stansbury FC. Pathogenesis of myopia-a new classification. Arch Ophthalmol. 1948; 39: 273-99.
Suzuki H. Observations on the intraocular changes associated with accommodation: an experimental study using radiographic technique. Exp Eye Res. 1973; 17: 119-28.
Suzuki H. Neuronal influence on the mechanical activity of the ciliary muscle. Br J Ophthalmol. 1983; 78: 591-7.
Tomlinson A, Phillips CI. Applanation tension and axial length of the eyeball. Br J Ophthalmol. 1970; 54: 548-53.
Tomlinson A, Phillips CI. Unequal axial length of eyeball and ocular tension. Acta Ophthalmol. 1972; 50: 872-6.
Troilo D, Gottlieb MD, Wallman J. Visual deprivation causes myopia in chicks with optic nerve section. Curr Eye Res. 1987; 6: 993-9.
Van Alphen GWHM. On emmetropia and ametropia. Ophthalmologica (Suppl). 1961; 142: 1-92.
Van Alphen GWHM. Choroidal stress and emmetropization. Vis Res. 1986; 26: 723-34.
Van Alphen GWHM. Emmetropization in the primate eye. In: Myopia and the Control of Eye Growth- Ciba Foundation Symposium. Chichester: John Wiley & Sons; 1990: 115-25.
Von Arlt. 1856. Cited in Donders FC. On the anomalies of accommodation and refraction of the eye. Trans. Moore WD. London: The New Sydenham Society. 1864; 447.
Von Arlt CF. Ueber die ursachen und die entstehung der kurzsichtigkeit. Vienna: Wilhelm Braumüller, 1876. Cited in Stansbury FC. Pathogenesis of myopia- a new classification. Arch Ophthalmol. 1948; 39: 273-99.
Von Graefe A. Beiträge zur physiologie und pathologie der schiefen augenmusckeln. Arch f Ophth. 1854; 1: 1-167.Cited in Stansbury FC. Pathogenesis of myopia-a new classification. Arch Ophthalmol. 1948; 39: 273-99.

Wallman J, Rosenthal D, Adams JI, Trachtman JN, Romagnano L. Role of accommodation and developmental aspects of experimental myopia in chicks. In: Fledelius HC, Alsbirk PH, Goldschmidt E, eds. Third International Conference on Myopia, Copenhagen. The Hague: Dr W. Junk Publishers. Doc Ophthalmol Proc Series. 1981; 28: 197-206.

Young FA. The effect of atropine on the development of myopia in monkeys. Am J Optom Arch Am Acad Optom. 1965; 42: 439-49.

Young FA. The development and control of myopia in human and subhuman primates. Contacto. 1975; 19: 16-31.

Young FA. The nature and control of myopia. J Am Optom Assoc. 1977; 48: 451-7.

Young FA. Intraocular pressure dynamics associated with accommodation. In: Fledelius HC, Alsbirk PH, Goldschmidt E, eds. Third International Conference on Myopia, Copenhagen. The Hague: Dr W. Junk Publishers. Doc Ophthalmol Proc Ser. 1981a; 28: 171-6.

Young FA. Primate myopia. Am J Optom Physiol Opt. 1981b; 58: 560-6.

Young FA, Leary GA. Accommodation and vitreous chamber pressure: a proposed mechanism for myopia. In: Grosvenor TP, Flom MC, eds. Refractive Anomalies. Boston: Butterworth-Heinemann; 1991: 301-9.

CHAPTER 6
RETINAL DEFOCUS AND MYOPIGENESIS

The association between specific altered visual input early in life and axial ocular growth in experimental animals as well as in humans has been of considerable interest over the past two decades (see Goss and Criswell 1981, Yinon 1984, Smith 1991, Chung 1993, Hung et al. 1995, Norton and Siegwart 1995, Edwards 1996 for reviews). Degradation of the retinal image occurs following certain congenital pathological conditions, as well as with certain experimental manipulations. In humans, congenital anomalies in the form of opacities in the ocular media, such as cataracts, or other conditions such as complete ptosis, deprive the eye of pattern vision. In animals, such form degradation/deprivation occurs following the introduction of high-powered lenses or lid suture, respectively. These specific alterations in early visual experience have been demonstrated to induce myopia, predominantly resulting from posterior chamber axial elongation. Local retinal factors in the regulation of axial growth have recently been invoked as possible trigger mechanisms (see Goss and Wickham 1995 for an excellent review). A brief overview of some of the relevant studies will be the focus of this chapter.

MONKEYS

In primates, Wiesel and Raviola (1977) induced monocular lid fusion at various times in young macaques and found a maximum interocular refractive difference of 13.5D, with the affected eye always being markedly myopic. Postmortem examination of the treated eye revealed an elongation of approximately 20% in the axial dimension and an increase of 7% in the equatorial diameter. The posterior sclera was thinner, while the cornea, choroid, and retinal thickness remained unaltered. Corneal refraction was not affected. Similar results were found using a binocular lid fusion paradigm, with up to 11D of myopia present in each eye. The absence of consistent changes in any of the other ocular components was confirmed in later studies using either similar lid suture techniques (Raviola and Wiesel 1985) or experimentally-induced corneal opacification (Wiesel and Raviola 1979). However, the effects of lid fusion were not apparent when the animals were raised in darkness (Raviola and Wiesel 1978). This important finding suggested that the myopia was due to the altered visual input rather than either the mechanical effects or changes in the anterior segment environmental conditions due to the closed lids themselves. Moreover, the myopization was suggested to be mediated through subcortical centers, since myopia could still be induced when the visual cortex was removed.

In contrast, monocular degradation of retinal focus produced by addition of a -9D contact lens resulted in 5 out of 8 rhesus monkeys developing axial hyperopia (Smith et al. 1994). Other studies using similar techniques for producing optical defocus resulted in either an absence of refractive changes or in relative axial hyperopia; no myopia was found (Crewther et al. 1988, Chung 1993, Bradley et al. 1996, Hung and Smith 1996, Lambert et al. 1996). In fact, Hung and Smith (1996) showed that hyperopia developed regardless of the direction of retinal defocus. It was thus postulated that severe forms of visual deprivation, such as in lid occlusion, lead to axial elongation, while less severe forms of image degradation, such as aphakia, lead to the retardation of axial growth (Bradley et al. 1996), at least in rhesus monkeys.

The role of accommodation in the development of myopia was addressed in later studies by Raviola and Wiesel (1985, 1990). Atropinization was performed, and its differential effect on form deprivation from that produced by lid fusion was found to vary with the species of the monkey. While atropine bore no effects on lid fusion-induced myopia in the rhesus monkey, it prevented axial elongation and correlated myopia in stumptailed monkeys. Therefore, the process of accommodation *per se* did not seem to play a role in inducing myopia in rhesus monkeys. In fact, removal of the ciliary ganglion or optic nerve section had no deterrent effect either. Hence, a local rather than a central mechanism apparently triggered by the lack of retinal-image contrast was implicated in the development of myopia in the rhesus monkey. However, here the role of accommodation was clearly species dependent.

CHICKS

Monocular and binocular lid closure in neonate chicks similarly produced myopia of greater than 6D in the treated eyes (Shapiro 1981). While the axial length was found to increase by approximately 2mm, Shapiro claimed that this did not fully account for the total increase in myopia, since keratometry revealed flattening of the cornea by as much as 5.82D. According to Shapiro, this flattening was due to enlargement of the globe. Shapiro further speculated that the lens may play a role, although no data were presented in support of this notion. Shapiro also suggested that the resultant myopia was not accommodatively-induced. Since an extremely poor quality, nearly contrastless retinal image was formed with complete lid closure, accommodation may not have been stimulated (Ciuffreda 1991). In agreement with studies on primates, Shapiro indicated that myopia was not a central cortical phenomenon, since the effects of both monocular and binocular lid closure were similar.

The non-central, more local nature of the induced myopia was also demonstrated by Wallman et al. (1987) (Figure 6-1). Neonate chicks received either complete (entire retina being affected) or partial (either temporal or nasal hemiretina being affected) form deprivation through the use of white translucent full or hemifield occluders, respectively, for a period of 2 to 6 weeks. Eyes receiving total deprivation became myopic throughout the entire retina. In contrast, eyes receiving partial deprivation exhibited "local" regions of myopia, i.e., only the visually-deprived region became myopic to a statistically significant degree, while the normally stimulated region remained nearly emmetropic. The induced myopia (median=-15D), whether global or local in nature, resulted from enlargement of the vitreous chamber in the corresponding region. *It was thus concluded that myopia cannot be the result of a global process such as increased intraocular pressure or accommodative biomechanics, but rather due to local regulation of vision-dependent ocular growth.*

The notion of myopia as a consequence of a local growth process also appeared to be supported by other findings. It was reported that deprivation myopia was still induced despite optic nerve section (Troilo et al. 1987, Wildsoet and Pettigrew 1988). More recent findings by Leech et al. (1995) have demonstrated that the intravitreal administration of pirenzepine, a muscarinic M_1 antagonist, was effective against the development of myopia and axial enlargement in monocularly form-deprived chicks. Pirenzepine was believed to act on the receptor sites located at the retinal or choroidal level, thus influencing the regulation of ocular growth.

More recently, Wallman et al. (1995) documented the role of the choroid in modulating the refractive error in vitro as well as in vivo chick eyes. As demonstrated in their earlier study (Wallman et al. 1987), either full-field or regional deprivation myopia was induced in chick eyes following the use of appropriate translucent diffusers. This was accounted for by elongation of the vitreous chamber in the deprived region. Upon cessation of the deprivation treatment and subsequent exposure to the normal visual environment, the affected part of the choroid was found to increase in thickness, apparently in an attempt to compensate for the induced myopia. This expansion of the choroid, which caused the retina to be shifted anteriorly, resulted in myopic reduction. In fact, it was reported that the time course of choroidal expansion paralleled the refractive change. In addition, the use of spectacle lenses also resulted in compensatory changes in choroidal thickness. Positive lenses which rendered the eye myopic caused the choroid to expand. Conversely, negative lenses which rendered the eye hyperopic caused subsequent thinning of the choroid. And, as in the diffuser paradigm described earlier, these choroidal effects were reversed upon removal of the lenses in the young animals.

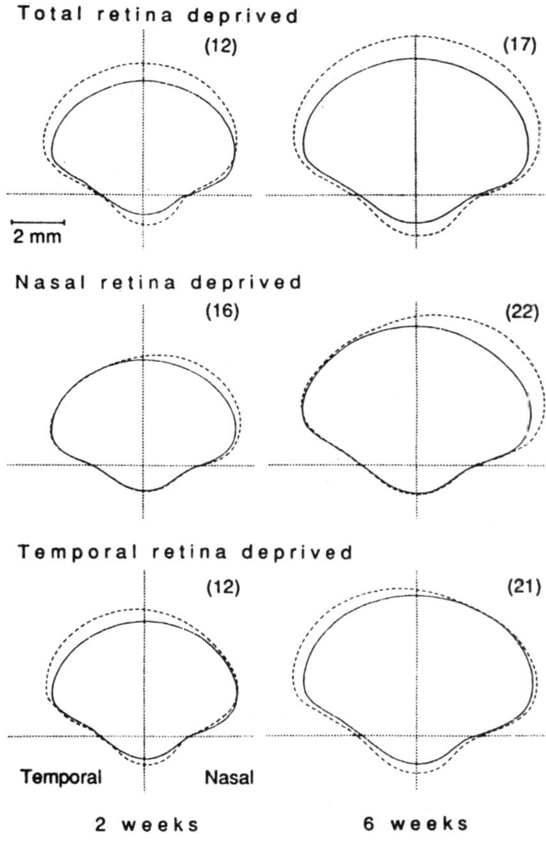

Figure 6-1 : Effects of visual deprivation on the shape of the eyes. Averages traced from photographs; the interrupted line is the deprived eye; the solid line is the control eye from the same animal. All eyes are presented as right eyes, viewed from above. The "optic axis" is defined here as the perpendicular bisecting the line joining the corneal margins (Reprinted with permission, Wallman et al. 1987).

Accommodation was also eliminated as a factor contributing to the development of myopia in a study by Schaeffel and associates (1990) in which marked anisometropia was artificially induced. The imposition of asymmetric interocular defocus with use of positive spherical lenses (+2 or +4D) in one eye and negative spherical lenses (-4 or -8D) in the fellow eye resulted in correspondingly short, hyperopic eyes and long, myopic eyes. Thus, eyes which were rendered artificially hyperopic or myopic grew appropriately in the axial dimension to compensate for the induced blur. This occurred despite the absence of accommodative function as a consequence of lesions to the Edinger-Westphal nuclei, thus supporting the previously stated notion that accommodation per se was not a necessary factor.

KITTENS

Less consistent results have been found in kittens. One technique used was the optical induction of anisometropia through the monocular introduction of negative lenses incorporated into goggles (Smith et al. 1980). Kittens were initially reared in darkness for 28 days followed by the introduction of the goggles. The control eye received plano power lenses, while the fellow eye received a high power negative lens (-10 to -16D) daily for 2 to 3 hours over a period of 2 months. At the conclusion of the test period, the eyes receiving plano treatment became hyperopic by +1.06D, while the deprived eyes became myopic by -1.12D. The majority of cases (5 out of 8) exhibited elongation of the deprived eye, with a high correlation between axial length and refractive change. The axial myopia was attributed to the defocused retinal image.

Form deprivation by monocular lid suture in neonates also produced a mean elongation of 1.37 mm in the treated eye (Kirby et al. 1982) due primarily to an increase in length of the posterior segment. While axial elongation was demonstrated in all animals, only half of them exhibited myopia with powers ranging from -0.50 to -3D. One-half also showed a tendency for the cornea to flatten to compensate for the increase in axial length. On the other hand, Gollender and Thorn (1979) reported inconsistent axial length changes. While the majority of kittens exhibited elongation, some exhibited shortening. The structural correlates were found in both the aqueous and vitreous chambers, while lens thickness remained constant.

In contrast, Nathan and associates (1984) were not able to replicate the above findings. Neither myopia nor axial length changes were observed following alteration of patterned vision, which was accomplished using either of the following methods: monocular or binocular introduction of high-powered rigid contact lenses, or monocular lid suture and monocular atropinization. No significant changes in the ocular dimensions were found as a result of either technique. These discrepancies were attributed to the visual experience prior to the inducement period, the methodology, i.e., the use of contact lenses versus goggles, and the length of the inducement period (Grosvenor 1989).

OTHER NON-HUMAN SPECIES

The resultant axial myopia induced by degradation of retinal-image contrast was documented not only in the aforementioned species, but other species as well, e.g., tree shrews (McKanna and Casagrande 1978a, 1978b, Marsh-Tootle and Norton 1989, McBrien and Norton 1992) and marmosets (Troilo 1996). Thus, it appeared to be a robust phenomenon.

HUMANS

Data from studies in humans subjected to anomalous pattern vision early in life resulting from a variety of ocular anomalies also support the hypothesis of form-deprivation induced myopia. Several relevant studies will be described below.

Gee and Tabbara (1988) examined 39 patients with either bilateral or unilateral corneal opacification occurring from birth through 64 years of age. In eyes with bilateral corneal opacities, the axial lengths were significantly increased as compared to age and sex-matched controls. Similarly, in eyes with unilateral corneal opacities, the axial lengths were significantly increased relative to the unaffected eyes. And, in the latter group, patients whose disease onset was prior to 7 years of age had significantly greater axial lengths than patients with later onset. This is consistent with the notion of age-related visual system susceptiblity to abnormal visual experience (Ciuffreda 1986, Ciuffreda et al. 1991).

Analogous to lid fusion studies in animals, unilateral ptosis in children has also resulted in a greater degree of myopia in the affected eye (O'Leary and Millodot 1979). Similar results were found in a retrospective study using data derived from ophthalmological as well as optometric practices (Rabin et al. 1981). The data consisted of patients who were exposed to various forms of anomalous pattern vision by virtue of pathological conditions affecting one or both eyes early in life. These included congenital cataracts, retrolental fibroplasia, congenital optic atrophy, and juvenile macular dystrophy. In all instances, myopia of at least -2.14D was found in the affected eye(s). In seven cases of monocular pattern deprivation, the affected eyes exhibited a significantly greater amount of myopia relative to their fellow eyes, with the interocular difference ranging from 5.50 to 12.25D. Ultrasonographic data on two additional subjects revealed abnormally increased axial lengths. The array of ocular anomalies reported in this study represented various forms of vision deprivation. Thus, the related myopization appears to be a general phenomenon. Exposure to anomalous pattern vision resulted in myopia irrespective of the nature of the deprivation. The myopia induced by altered visual input early in life was undeniably a consequence of an increase in axial length. Similar findings were reported by Nathan et al. (1985), whose population also included nystagmats.

In another study, Hoyt et al. (1981) reported unilateral axial myopia associated with unilateral neonatal eyelid closure. The closure was due to various ocular anomalies, e.g., blepharoptosis, congenital third nerve palsy, and swelling of periorbital structures. The myopia ranged from -4.25 to -7D as compared with refractive errors ranging from +1.75 to -0.50D (spherical equivalent) in the fellow eye. While no significant interocular asymmetry was found with respect to corneal power, anterior segment depth, or lens thickness, the vitreous length was consistently and significantly larger in the myopic eye, with this difference ranging from 1.6 to 2.8mm. The increase in vitreal chamber depth effectively accounted for all of the induced refractive difference. Axial elongation in the affected eyes was further confirmed in the majority of patients with either unilateral (von Noorden and Lewis 1987, Rasooly and BenEzra 1988) or bilateral (Rasooly and BenEzra 1988) cataract or aphakia early in life. Unilateral form deprivation myopia was also reported by Johnson et al. (1982) in their investigation of a case of congenital lens opacity affecting one of a pair of identical twins. While the non-deprived eye of one twin exhibited similar refraction, visual acuity, and axial length as the other twin, the deprived eye was more myopic by over 6D. Visual acuity was markedly reduced, and the axial length was 2mm longer, in the highly myopic eye.

Lastly, there is debate with regard to the use of full myopic correction. Some feel that undercorrection at distance resulting in a reduced accommodative demand at near slows myopic progression (Angle and Wissmann 1980), whereas others believe it may interrupt the natural emmetropization process (Medina 1987a,b, Hung et al, 1995). However, recent evidence suggests that full myopic correction in very young children (1 1/2 - 4 1/2 years of age) does not exacerbate myopic progression. In fact, it was strongly suggested that undercorrection not be used, as this would introduce increased amounts of retinal defocus that are myopigenic in nature (Angi et al. 1996). Clearly, the proper amount of correction for myopia remains a controversial topic, especially with regard to young children.

SUMMARY

The common element in the majority of studies using different species, including humans, and diverse techniques appeared to be the alteration of the visual input, more specifically, degradation of the retinal image during the early critical developmental period. The resultant optical defocus/reduced contrast acted as a trigger mechanism for the induction of axial myopia. However, it should be emphasized that the full and direct application of animal models to human myopia should be exercised with some caution, since distinct differences do exist (Zadnik and Mutti 1995, Edwards 1996), even within the same species (Raviola and Wiesel 1985, 1990).

REFERENCES

Angi MR, Forattini F, Segalla C, Mantovani E. Myopia evolution in pre-school children after full optical correction. Strabismus 1996; 4: 145-57.

Angle J, Wissmann DA. Myopia and corrective lenses. Soc Sci Med. 1980; 14A: 473-9.

Bradley DV, Fernandes A, Tigges M, Boothe RG. Diffuser contact lenses retard axial elongation in infant rhesus monkeys. Vis Res. 1996; 36: 509-14.

Chung KM. Critical review: effects of optical defocus on refractive development and ocular growth and relation to accommodation. Optom Vis Sci. 1993; 70: 228-33.
Ciuffreda KJ. Accommodation and its anomalies. In: Charman WN, ed. Vision and Visual Dysfunction, vol. 1 (Visual Optics and Instrumentation). London: MacMillan; 1991: 237-79.
Ciuffreda KJ. Visual system plasticity in human amblyopia. In: Hilfer SR, Sheffield JB, eds. Development of Order in the Visual System. New York: Springer-Verlag; 1986: 211-44.
Ciuffreda KJ, Levi DM, Selenow A. Amblyopia: Basic and Clinical Aspects. Boston: Butterworths; 1991.
Crewther SG, Nathan J, Kiely PM, Brennan NA, Crewther DP. The effect of defocussing contact lenses on refraction in cynomolgus monkeys. Clin Vis Sci. 1988; 3: 221-8.
Edwards MH. Animal models of myopia. Acta Ophthalmol Scand. 1996; 74: 213-9.
Gee SS, Tabbara KF. Increase in ocular axial length in patients with corneal opacification. Ophthalmol. 1988; 95: 1276-8.
Gollender M, Thorn F. Development of axial ocular dimensions following eyelid suture in the cat. Vis Res. 1979; 19: 221-3.
Goss DA, Criswell MH. Myopia development in experimental animal—literature review. Am J Optom. 1981; 58: 859-69.
Goss DA, Wickham MG. Retinal-image mediated ocular growth as a mechanism for juvenile onset myopia and for emmetropization. Doc Ophthalmol. 1995; 90: 341-75.
Grosvenor T. Myopia and its development. In: Primary Care Optometry. New York: Professional Press Books/Fairchild Publications; 1989: 57-89.
Hoyt CS, Stone RD, Fromer C, Billson FA. Monocular axial myopia associated with neonatal eyelid closure in human infants. Am J Ophthalmol. 1981; 91: 197-200.
Hung LF, Crawford MLJ, Smith EL III. Spectacle lenses alter eye growth and the refractive status of young monkeys. Nature Med. 1995; 1: 761-5.
Hung LF, Smith EL III. Extended wear, soft, contact lenses produce hyperopia in young monkeys. Optom Vis Sci. 1996; 579-84.
Johnson CA, Post RB, Chalupa LM, Lee TJ. Monocular deprivation in humans: a study of identical twins. Invest Ophthalmol Vis Sci. 1982; 23: 135-8.
Kirby AW, Sutton L, Weiss H. Elongation of cat eyes following neonatal lid suture. Invest Ophthalmol Vis Sci. 1982; 22: 274-7.
Lambert SR, Fernandes A, Drews-Botsch C, Tigges M. Pseudophakia retards axial elongation in neonatal monkey eyes. Invest Ophthalmol Vis Sci. 1996; 37: 451-8.
Leech EM, Cottriall CL, McBrien NA. Pirenzepine prevents form deprivation myopia in a dose dependent manner. Ophthal Physiol Opt. 1995; 15: 351-6.
Marsh-Tootle WL, Norton TT. Refractive and structural measures of lid-suture myopia in tree shrews. Invest Ophthalmol Vis Sci. 1989; 30: 2245-57.
McBrien NA, Norton TT. The development of experimental myopia and ocular component dimensions in monocularly lid-sutured tree shrews (Tupaia Belangeri). Vis Res. 1992; 32: 843-52.
McKanna JA, Casagrande VA. Reduced lens development in lid-sutured myopia. Exp Eye Res. 1978a; 26: 715-23.
McKanna JA, Casagrande VA. Zonular dysplasia in myopia. Proc Second International Conference on Myopia. Sato T, Yamaji R, eds. Yokohama 1978b; 21-32.
Medina A. A model for emmetropization—predicting the progression of ametropia. Ophthalmol. 1987a; 194: 133-9.
Medina A. A model for emmetropization- the effect of corrective lenses. Acta Ophthalmol. 1987b; 65: 565-71.
Nathan J, Crewther SG, Crewther DP, Kiely PM. Effects of retinal image degradation on ocular growth in cats. Invest Ophthalmol Vis Sci. 1984; 25: 1300-6.

Nathan J, Kiely PM, Crewther SG, Crewther DP. Disease-associated visual image degradation and spherical refractive errors in children. Am J Optom Physiol Opt. 1985; 62: 680-8.
Norton TT, Siegwart JT Jr. Animal models of emmetropization: matching axial length to the focal plane. J Am Optom Assoc.1995; 66: 405- 14.
O'Leary DJ, Millodot M. Eyelid closure causes myopia in humans. Experientia. 1979; 35: 1478-9.
Rabin J, Van Sluyters RC, Malach R. Emmetropization: a vision-dependent phenomenon. Invest Ophthalmol Vis Sci. 1981; 20: 561-4.
Rasooly R, BenEzra D. Congenital and traumatic cataract: the effect on ocular axial growth. Arch Ophthalmol. 1988; 106: 1066-8.
Raviola E, Wiesel TN. Effect of dark rearing on experimental myopia in monkeys. Invest Ophthalmol Vis Sci. 1978; 17: 485-8.
Raviola E, Wiesel TN. An animal model of myopia. New Engl J Med. 1985; 312: 1609-15.
Raviola E, Wiesel TN. Neural control of eye growth and experimental myopia in primates. In: Myopia and the Control of Eye Growth- Ciba Foundation Symposium. Chichester: John Wiley & Sons; 1990: 22-44.
Schaeffel F, Troilo D, Wallman J, Howland HC. Developing eyes that lack accommodation grow to compensate for imposed defocus. Vis Neurosci. 1990; 4: 177-83.
Shapiro A. Experimental visual deprivation and myopia. In: Fledelius HC, Alsbirk PH, Goldschmidt E, eds. Third International Conference on Myopia. The Hague: Dr W. Junk Publishers; 1981: 193-5.
Smith EL III. Experimentally induced refractive anomalies in mammals. In: Grosvenor T, Flom MC, eds. Refractive Anomalies—Research and Clinical Applications. Boston: Butterworth-Heinemann; 1991: 246-67.
Smith EL III, Hung LF, Harwerth RS. Effects of optically induced blur on the refractive status of young monkeys. Vis Res. 1994; 34: 293-301.
Smith EL III, Maguire GW, Watson JT. Axial lengths and refractive errors in kittens reared with an optically induced anisometropia. Invest Ophthalmol Vis Sci. 1980; 19: 1250 -5.
Troilo D. Effects of form deprivation myopia on retinal anatomy and cone distribution in the common marmoset. Invest Ophthalmol Vis Sci (Suppl). 1996; 37: 323.
Troilo D, Gottlieb MD, Wallman J. Visual deprivation causes myopia in chicks with optic nerve section. Curr Eye Res. 1987; 6: 993-9.
Von Noorden GK, Lewis RA. Ocular axial length in unilateral congenital cataracts and blepharoptosis. Invest Ophthalmol Vis Sci. 1987; 28: 750-2.
Wallman J, Gottlieb MD, Rajaram V, Fugate-Wentzek LA. Local retinal regions control local eye growth and myopia. Science. 1987; 237: 73-7.
Wallman J, Wildsoet C, Xu A, Gottlieb MD, Nickla D, Marran L, Krebs W, Christensen AM. Moving the retina: choroidal modulation of the refractive state. Vis Res. 1995; 35: 37-50.
Wiesel TN, Raviola E. Myopia and eye enlargement after neonatal lid fusion in monkeys. Nature (Lond). 1977; 266: 66-8.
Wiesel TN, Raviola E. Increase in axial length of the macaque monkey eye after corneal opacification. Invest Ophthalmol Vis Sci. 1979; 18: 1232-6.
Wildsoet CF, Pettigrew JD. Experimental myopia and anomalous eye growth patterns unaffected by optic nerve section in chicks: evidence for local control of eye growth. Clin Vis Sci. 1988; 3: 99-107.
Yinon U. Myopia induction in animals following alteration of the visual input during development: a review. Curr Eye Res. 1984; 3: 677-90.
Zadnik K, Mutti DO. How applicable are animal myopia models to human juvenile onset myopia. Vis Res. 1995; 35: 1283-8.

CHAPTER 7
MYOPIA: PAST, PRESENT AND FUTURE

LACK OF SIGNIFICANT BIOMECHANICAL EFFECTS OF ACCOMMODATION AND CONVERGENCE ON MYOPIGENESIS

Over the past several decades, there has been considerable experimental and theoretical work investigating the biomechanical contributions of accommodation and convergence on the tunics of the eye, especially the choroid and sclera, with regard to their role in the development of myopia. However, as discussed in Chapter 5, their impact appears to be minimal at best.

There are several arguments that frequently are presented in this literature that appear to be misleading, or at least have been misinterpreted. First, there is one theory of accommodation which advocates that the vitreous body plays a major biomechanical role in accommodation (Coleman 1970). However, the unique report of Fisher (1983) casts serious doubt on it. He demonstrated that the monocular amplitude of accommodation was the same (~9D) in each eye of a young adult patient who had a complete unilateral vitrectomy. However, there was more response variability in the vitrectomized eye, which suggests that the gelatinous vitreous body may serve to provide a modest degree of stability to the lens during marked accommodation when the zonules are least taut, and the lens is therefore susceptible to small and transient internal and external forces and related perturbations. Second, the comparison is often made that the maximal force of contraction of the intraocular ciliary muscles is only 0.5g, whereas that of the extraocular muscles may be as high as 150g. Of course, such comparisons are only valid when the biomechanical aspects of the object being acted upon are considered. A force of 0.5g acting on the highly elastic choroid is quite sufficient to stretch it readily. A force of 150g (which is quite non-naturalistic) might have impact upon the tough fibrous sclera. However, the extraocular muscle forces are typically less than 40g under most naturalistic conditions. And, if one now considers the mechanical stress of oblique muscle contraction on the posterior sclera, it typically does not exceed 4g (Greene 1991). Such a relatively small force is of little consequence on the sclera. Third, and lastly, arguments have been made and data presented indicating that during increased accommodation, the pressure in the vitreous chamber increases by approximately 2mm Hg. However, the pressure in the suprachoroidal space adjacent to the sclera concurrently *decreases* 1mm Hg or so. In addition, the vitreous force is distributed throughout the eye, and therefore it would have little differential impact on the posterior region of the eye (Goss and Wickham 1995).

RETINAL DEFOCUS AND MYOPIGENESIS

Over the past twenty years or so, there has been a growing body of evidence suggesting the rather unique proposition that retinal defocus and the correlated retinal image contrast degradation are responsible for producing the subsequent change in axial length (see Chapters 4 and 6). This has been attributed to local biochemical alterations in the sclera and related contiguous ocular structures (see Goss and Wickham 1995 for a detailed review). The imposed retinal defocus was typically large and constant in nature, with it being created by introduction of high powered spherical lenses.

Although the resultant change in axial length was frequently direction specific such that it served to reduce the newly-created refractive error, i.e., it produced emmetropization, this has not always been the case even in primates (Smith et al. 1994, Hung and Smith 1996). However, this may not be surprising when one considers the nature of a pure blur input. It is an "even-error" signal. That is, the signal provides magnitude *but not* directional information about the system error (Stark 1968). Anyone who has conducted dynamic accommodation experiments using a Badal optical system in which only changes in blur (i.e., the stimulus to accommodation; Ciuffreda 1991) drives the system, and non-predictable stimuli such as randomized steps are employed, the *initial* accommodative response frequently occurs in the *wrong* direction. Only once the increased blur is perceived does the response alter direction to follow the true target direction (see Chapter 1). This directional ambiguity is especially true for small blur inputs as may be the case with NITM.

Could a similar process be implicated in the onset and/or progression of myopia? We believe this might be the case. There is considerable evidence demonstrating that the steady-state accommodative response in myopic eyes (even *before* they become myopic; see later discussion in this chapter) is slightly reduced at near (see Chapter 2). This would result in a slightly larger amount of retinal defocus (*not* necessarily producing the perception of blur, assuming the retinal image of the target remains within the eye's depth-of-focus), as the "lag of accommodation" would be increased. If near focus is sustained, the process of accommodative adaptation would eventually bias accommodation inward slightly, thus reducing the residual accommodative error a bit over time. However, when subsequently focusing at far, there would now also be increased accommodative error (i.e., NITM), especially in more susceptible individuals such as myopes. Therefore, *at both distance and near,* there would be a transient increase in retinal defocus with its potential myopigenic aspects, especially if one conceptualizes this process to be cumulative over time. In addition, it could result in pseudomyopia, which may also be a transitional factor in the development of permanent, axial-based myopia (see Chapters 3 and 4).

However, there is a potential problem with this argument. While the resultant retinal defocus at near is directionally appropriate to initiate myopic changes, at far it is not. At present, we believe that these very small amounts of retinal defocus associated with the subtle accommodative dysfunctions found in many myopic eyes may not be sufficient to provide directional information. All small amounts of retinal defocus would therefore always produce axial elongation. Our speculation will require confirmation from future human and animal studies.

NEARWORK-INDUCED TRANSIENT MYOPIA

The classic experiment of Lancaster and Williams (1914) over 80 years ago demonstrated clearly and quantitatively the phenomenon of "nearwork-induced transient myopia" (NITM) (see Chapter 4). However, only relatively recently has it resurfaced with its potential clinical importance as related to asthenopia and myopia due to the increased use of computers both at work and in the home. Ehrlich (1987) was the first to demonstrate NITM objectively. Under rather extreme binocular viewing conditions, a relatively small but significant amount of NITM was induced, and it *persisted* under normal distance binocular viewing conditions for at least 1 hour. This demontrated an inability to relax the ciliary muscle fully and rapidly upon subsequent gaze into the distance. One could speculate that perhaps if this cycle were repeated many times over a period of weeks or months in particularly susceptible individuals, a resultant pseudomyopia might develop. This could produce up to 1 diopter or so of refractive change (Stoddard, 1942). The unsuspecting and less experienced eye doctor might prescribe concave lenses for distance wear. However, the more experienced and probing practitioner might suspect that it was related to nearwork, especially if increased nearwork were being performed, and the symptom was intermittent rather than constant blur in the distance. Such a patient could be managed best by appropriate accommodative vision therapy and related techniques to reestablish normal static and dynamic accommodative (and interactive vergence) responsivity.

In our own laboratory, we have been conducting experiments in this area for the past 5 years or so. Before that, we (and others) had been investigating both tonic accommodation and accommodative adaptation to determine how they were influenced by nearwork and manipulation of various stimulus parameters, such as target distance and duration. The results were mixed (see Rosenfield et al. 1993, 1994 for reviews). See Chapter 4. However, these two parameters are measured in the dark (Figure 4-9). We thought that it might be more informative to determine how nearwork might influence the distance refractive state under naturalistic viewing *and* test conditions, and thus our shift to the NITM paradigm in which all tasks and measurements are obtained under normal illumination. The NITM results are summarized below (also see Chapter 4):

- both early- and late-onset myopes were most susceptible (Ciuffreda and Wallis, in preparation); most emmetropes and hyperopes were not.
- the response was blur-dominated (Ong and Ciuffreda 1995, Ong 1996, Ong et al, in preparation); it was little affected by either the vergence and/or proximal accommodative contributions (Rosenfield et al. 1992a, Ong et al, in preparation).
- it could be induced by as little as 4 minutes of nearwork (Ciuffreda et al. 1996).
- it demonstrated saturation at near, with its magnitude being the same for the 3 and 5 diopter accommodative stimulus levels tested (Ciuffreda et al. 1996).
- it could be reduced or prevented by taking frequent rest periods during the nearwork task (Rosenfield et al. 1992b).
- it could be prevented by wearing a near add equal to the accommodative stimulus level (Rosenfield et al. 1992b, Rosenfield 1994).
- when tested over a continuous 4-hour period of reading, some individuals (i.e., the emmetropes) showed no effect, whereas others (i.e., the myopes) demonstrated either a very brief or a sustained effect which suggested differing levels of nearwork susceptibility (Ciuffreda et al, in preparation).
- it was largest in magnitude with slowest decay and greatest variability in individuals who complained of transient distance blur following a short period of nearwork (Ciuffreda and Ordoñez, 1995).
- it could be reversed and was responsive to conventional optometric accommodative vision therapy (Ciuffreda and Ordoñez, in preparation).

What do our results suggest? It appears that for the more susceptible myope, even short durations of nearwork, presumably producing nearwork-induced retinal defocus/blur, may have both potential short- (Ong and Ciuffreda 1995) and long-term (Parssinen et al. 1993) consequences with respect to the distance refractive state. Furthermore, its effect on distance refraction may be prevented, reduced, and/or treated with use of relatively high near adds, regular rest intervals, and/or conventional optometric accommodative vision therapy. Our findings have the greatest potential impact on young children who are either "at risk" of developing myopia or who have just begun to develop their myopia. Our NITM paradigm could be adopted clinically either with use of dynamic retinoscopy to assess the pre/post-task refractive state directly or threshold visual acuity changes to assess it indirectly (Ong and Ciuffreda 1995) (see Chapter 4). And, the findings of Goss (1991b), Goss and Jackson (1996a) and Gwiazda and colleagues (1995) which demonstrated changes in specific accommodative and related measures either before or approximately concurrent with the development of myopia, respectively, forces us as optometrists to be more aggressive and creative in the implementation of appropriate preventive and treatment measures. Since the cost to society for refractive examinations and related optical appliances is estimated to be 4.6 billion dollars annually (Javitt and Chiang 1994), development of such measures can have tremendous impact on our patients as well as society at large (Table 7.1). Clearly, this route is far superior to refractive surgery with its high costs ($2000/eye), possible side effects (refractive instability for 18 months, glare problems, initial pain, infection, etc.), and residual refractive error (McDonnell, 1995).

TABLE 7-1

FACT SHEET ON REFRACTION AND MYOPIA (1990)

- 50% of the U.S. population wears spectacles or contact lenses
- 8 billion dollars were spent on vision care products
- 50 million primary care eye examinations were performed by optometrists
- 12 million primary care eye examinations were performed by ophthalmologists
- 20-25% of the U.S. population was myopic; thus, there were roughly 50 million myopes
- 4.6 billion dollars were spent (direct and indirect costs) related to myopic correction

(Data from Javitts and Chiang 1994)

Some recent important new results have also shed light in this area. Mei and Rong (1994) found that frank pseudomyopia *preceded* the development of permanent myopia in a relatively large percentage of young children tested in China. Thus, at least for some, pseudomyopia of nearwork origin may represent a *transitional* phase between emmetropia and the onset of permanent myopia. Use of cycloplegic refraction as an additional clinical tool in this population is clearly critical in the diagnosis. Furthermore, it serves as a baseline of comparison for all subsequent refractive changes. Thus, a detailed case history with attention to myopic risk factors such as the parent's refraction, nearwork habits, etc., cycloplegic refraction, careful vision examination with emphasis on near testing, and patient education to explain the preventive aspects of vision care appear to be reasonable initial guidelines for handling this important area of optometry.

CLINICAL PROFILE OF THE MYOPIC EYE

The myopic eye can be characterized by the following profile:

Increased vitreous chamber/axial length. Increased vitreous chamber (Tokoro and Kabe 1964, Francois and Goes 1969, Gernet 1981, Otsuka et al. 1981, Curtin 1985, Grosvenor and Scott 1993, 1994) and overall axial length (Stenstrom 1947, van Alphen 1961, Francois and Goes 1969, Fledelius 1981, Gernet 1981, Otsuka et al. 1981, Garner et al. 1990, Bullimore et al. 1992, Grosvenor and Scott 1993, Fledelius 1995) have been consistently found in myopes. This was true for both early- and late-onset myopes (Adams 1987, McBrien and Millodot 1987, Grosvenor and Scott 1991, Adams and McBrien 1992, Grosvenor 1994, Jiang and Woessner 1996). These changes occurred concurrent with the onset and subsequent progression of myopia (Mei and Rong 1994, Goss and Jackson 1995).

While changes have also been reported with respect to the other ocular components, the majority of studies have demonstrated that axial elongation is the primary mechanism invovled in the development of permanent myopia (Stenstrom 1948, van Alphen 1961, Grosvenor and Scott 1993). This elongation was primarily accounted for by an increase in vitreal chamber depth (Gernet 1981, McBrien and Millodot 1987).

Increased keratometric power. While the data strongly support the notion that increased axial length is the primary determinant of myopia, some studies have also reported increased corneal power in myopes. This was predominantly noted in high myopes (>-5D) (Baldwin 1962, Scott and Grosvenor 1993, 1994), while low myopes (<-4D) manifested corneal flattening (Baldwin 1962). On the other hand, Harrie (1987) found that in low degrees of myopia (<-1.50D), the corneal curvature contributed substantially to the overall myopia, while for greater amounts of myopia (>-1.50D), the axial length was the single most important factor. Increased corneal power was also believed by some to be the basis for late-onset myopia (Kent 1963, Grosvenor and Scott 1991), as well as myopic progression during young adulthood but not during childhood (Sorsby and Leary 1970, Goss et al. 1985, Goss and Erickson 1987, Goss 1991a), with the rate of corneal change accounting for approximately one-half of the total myopic change (Goss et al. 1985). Based on these studies, Goss (1991a) concluded that early-onset myopia was primarily axial in nature, whereas the development of late-onset myopia was attributed at least in part to the cornea. However, according to Grosvenor and Scott (1991, 1993), this apparent distinction between early and late-onset myopes was not directly associated with the age of onset of the myopia but rather its degree. In addition, while corneal steepening was noted to correspond with the development of late-onset myopia, the primary change still occurred in the vitreous chamber length (Adams and McBrien 1992).

However, corneal steepening has been a less consistent finding (Sorsby et al. 1957, Baldwin 1962, Sorsby and Leary 1970, Goss and Jackson 1992, 1995). Most studies did not find a significant difference in either corneal curvature or power between refractive subgroups (Donders 1864, Sorsby et al. 1962a, Baldwin 1964, 1965, Tokoro and Kabe 1964, Franceschetti and Luyckx 1966, Francois and Goes 1969, Gernet 1981, Garner et al. 1992), nor between each eye of anisometropes (Francois and Goes 1969, Otsuka et al. 1981). Thus, the corneal contribution to myopic changes remains a point of some debate.

Increased axial length/corneal radius ratio (AL/CR). Increased AL/CR was noted by some investigators (Goss and Jackson 1992, Grosvenor and Scott 1994, Goss and Jackson 1995). The AL/CR ratio was found to be approximately 3 for emmetropes and significantly greater than 3 for myopes. This supports the notion that the resultant refractive status depends on the correlation of the ocular components. It also suggests that any increase in axial length that is not compensated by a corresponding flattening of the corneal curvature would result in myopia. And lastly, it can be of clinical predictive value as discussed later.

Flatter lens curvature/reduced lens power. This was reported by several investigators (Tron 1929, Stenstrom 1946, 1947, 1948, Sato 1957, Tokoro and Kabe 1964, Franceschetti and Gernet 1965a,b, Franceschetti and Luyckx 1966, Francois and Goes 1969, Gernet 1981, Garner et al. 1992, Grosvenor and Scott 1993). It was also reported in late-onset myopes (McBrien and Millodot 1987). This reduced lens power was believed to be compensatory in nature with respect to the increased axial change in myopic eyes (Franceschetti and Gernet 1965a, Francois and Goes 1969, Harrie 1987, Garner et al. 1992, Sorsby 1994). This is consistent with the proposal that the lens is the primary component responsible for the emmetropization process (Franceschetti and Gernet 1965a). In contrast, some studies have reported either increased lens power in myopes or no consistent relation between either lens thickness or lens power and refractive status (Tron 1929, Sorsby and Leary 1970, Larsen 1971b, Storey et al. 1990, Grosvenor and Scott 1991, 1994), as well as between each eye of anisometropes (Otsuka et al. 1981). Thus, further careful work is required to answer this important question. Comprehensive biometric measures performed longitudinally in a large group of children who are still emmetropic but at risk of becoming myopic should be studied.

Deeper anterior chamber depth. Increased anterior chamber depth was observed in myopes (Francois and Goes 1969, Larsen 1971a, Fledelius 1981, Storey et al. 1990, Grosvenor and Scott 1991), including late-onset myopes (McBrien and Millodot 1987). However, the anterior chamber depth differences between refractive groups were extremely small in magnitude [~0.1-0.2mm, with it being approximately equivalent to 0.20 to 0.40D (Erickson 1977)]. Its impact paled in comparison to the differences found for the other ocular components. Once again, along with a flatter lens, increased anterior chamber depth was suggested to be related to emmetropization, with the general effect of reducing overall refractive power (McBrien and Millodot 1987).

A firm knowledge of the normative values and their ranges in emmetropes for the various ocular parameters clearly has predictive value and may serve as a useful diagnostic and prognostic clinical tool. However, relative rather than absolute values should be considered, since biometric data have exhibited a wide range of inter- and intra-refractive group variability (Tron 1940, Sorsby et al. 1957, 1962a). For example, axial length varied from 20 to 27mm in emmetropes, 21 to 25mm in hyperopes, and a still wider range of 22 to 38mm in myopes (Tron 1940). Hence, it is not unlikely that some ametropic eyes would exhibit values falling within the emmetropic range and vice versa.

Increased intraocular pressure. Intraocular pressure was reported to be increased in myopes (Abdalla and Hamdi 1970, Tomlinson and Phillips 1970, Barraquer 1974, David et al. 1985, Pruett 1988, Edwards and Brown 1993). See Chapter 5 for a more detailed discussion. While elevated intraocular pressure had long been hypothesized to be the underlying factor in axial myopia, nonetheless, as discussed in Chapter 5, much of the data would not be consistent with this notion. Firstly, intraocular pressure in myopes was only slightly elevated (generally by 2 mm Hg or so) and was thus within the normal diurnal variation of intraocular pressure (Duke-Elder 1952, Drance 1960, Phelps et al. 1974). Secondly, investigations on the biomechanical aspects of intraocular pressure on the globe suggested that rather than being the precursor, the increased intraocular pressure may in fact have been the consequence of an axially elongated eye (Tomlinson and Phillips 1970, 1972). In fact, Edwards and Brown (1996) recently reported that this small increase in intraocular pressure did not occur until *after* the eye became myopic.

Reduced scleral rigidity. Scleral rigidity was found to be significantly less in myopes (Castrén and Pohjola 1961). This did not appear to be related to any unique structural properties characterizing myopic eyes, but rather to their increased eye size (Perkins 1981b).

Structural and biochemical changes in the myopic sclera. Myopic scleras exhibited a number of structural changes. These included narrowing and dissociation of the collagen fiber bundles, increased extensibility, increased prevalence of stellate fibrils, a preponderance of fibril groups with extremely fine diameters (Curtin and Teng 1958, Curtin et al. 1979), a predominantly lamellar collagen architecture, reduced fibril diameter, greater range of fibril diameters (Curtin and Teng 1958, Curtin et al. 1979, Liu et al. 1986), severe thinning (Curtin and Teng 1958, Curtin et al. 1979, Avetisov et al. 1984, Cheng et al. 1992), reduced collagen content (Avetisov et al. 1984), and disrupted or "splayed" fibers at the posterior sclera (Curtin and Teng 1958). In addition, myopic eyes also exhibited reduced content of hexosamines in the posterior sclera, as well as increased acid and neutral salt soluble collagen (Avetisov et al. 1984). These differences in scleral structure and hence its functional properties translate into a relatively weakened sclera and suggest a structural breakdown of the scleral collagen. In fact, tensile strength in myopic eyes was less than in emmetropic eyes, and it closely resembled that of the "at risk" group which was characterized by a mechanically weaker sclera (Avetisov et al. 1984). In non-human species, the biochemical composition of form-deprived myopic eyes was also altered (Norton and Rada 1995). This included a reduced level of sulfated glycosaminoglycans, reduced hydroxyproline, reduced sulfated glycosaminoglycan:DNA ratio, reduced glycosaminoglycan:hydroxyproline ratio, and reduced accumulation of collagen at the posterior pole. It was further suggested that the decreased extracellular matrix reduced scleral resistance (Norton and Rada 1995) and caused the myopic sclera to respond differently than eyes of the other refractive groups to similar amounts of stress (Phillips and McBrien 1995), therefore predisposing the eye to elongation (Norton and Rada 1995). However, since these changes were observed in eyes that were already myopic, it is not clear whether the morphological differences were the cause or the consequence of myopic development. Therefore, testing should be conducted during the entire course of experimental visual deprivation to determine the sequence of structural collagen and related biochemical changes in the eye and their relation to refractive state and axial length.

Structural changes in the myopic choroid and retina. Considerably thinner choroid and retina in myopes were revealed in cross-sectional measurements of the ocular coats (Mawas 1934). Mean values obtained were 0.8 mm for the normal and 0.25 mm for the highly myopic eyes. Such a variation in thickness alone yields a difference in stress by a factor of three for myopic eyes. This factor, in conjunction with those mentioned earlier, subject the myopic eye to a comparatively greater amount of mechanical stress than either emmetropic or hyperopic eyes. However, the actual impact of such added stress appears to be minimal.

Accommodation differences. Several accommodative parameters have been shown to be different in myopes. See Chapter 2 for details. Characteristics of blur-induced accommodation in myopes, which appear to be of relevance to the topic of myopigenesis, is considered below.

Accommodation has long been regarded as a potential myopigenic factor. As such, it has been suggested that any abnormal accommodation or accommodation at variance with that of emmetropes could act as a precursor for myopic development and progression. The overall finding from studies conducted with this aim in mind demonstrated a general trend for myopes to exhibit reduced accommodation at near. Moreover, this reduction was reported to be exaggerated under negative lens-induced blur paradigms in contrast to real target conditions (Gwiazda et al. 1993b). It was suggested that the reduced myopic accommodative responsivity might relate to a parallel reduction in blur sensitivity. What are the ramifications of reduced accommodative responsivity? During the performance of nearwork, this would translate into an accommodative lag greater than that normally encountered. The increased accommodative lag would result in an increased amount of retinal defocus. Since myopia had been linked to nearwork, greater amounts of sustained nearwork would result in a more or less persistent state of defocus. As the retinal defocus hypothesis suggests, over time this nearwork-induced chronic defocus may then act as a potential trigger mechanism in myopic development and progression by producing axial elongation (Goss 1991a, Held et al. 1994). More specifically, the greater lag observed in myopes for increasing amounts of accommodation results in a larger hyperopic defocus, i.e., the image is focused further behind the retinal plane. Hence, maximal retinal image clarity at near that can normally be achieved with appropriate accommodation may now be compensated with growth of the posterior segment. In essence, both accommodation and myopia serve the same function of ensuring retinal-image clarity (Goss 1991a, Gwiazda et al. 1995).

However, most of these deficits in accommodation and their effects on ocular growth were based on findings from subjects who were already myopic at the outset, and hence do not necessarily reflect the true sequence and correction of changes between accommodation and refractive status. Unfortunately, the results favoring pre-myopic changes appear to be mixed.

Both Goss (1991b) and Drobe and Saint-André (1995) presented convincing evidence for pre-myopic accommodative changes as discussed in the next section. In contrast, Gwiazda et al. (1995) reported that the reduced blur-driven accommodative response typically found in myopes did not precede the development of myopia, but rather occurred concurrent with myopic onset. Then, following the onset and upon slowed progression and stabilization of the myopia, an improvement of the accommodative response was observed albeit not fully normalized. However, since there was at least a 6-12 month time lag between measurements, any sudden transient or short-term changes might not have been detected; furthermore, with such relatively large temporal lags, the exact timing of events cannot be precise. Thus, longitudinal studies with shorter time intervals between measurements would be optimal in determining, with greater temporal resolution, the time course of these changes. Also, examining the response profile of potential myopes or those at risk for myopia might actually be more informative than those who are already myopic.

CLINICAL PREDICTORS OF MYOPIA

Several clinical parameters in pre-myopes were investigated in an attempt to ascertain more specifically the accommodative and vergence characteristics that may play a role in myopigenesis. It was hoped that these findings might have clinical predictive value. Ideally, if one could predict the development of myopia *prior* to its actual onset by identifying specific risk factors, then perhaps timely and appropriate intervention could be undertaken either to prevent the occurrence or at least reduce the final magnitude of myopia. Parameters that characterize the young pre-myopic profile include the following:

- less hyperopic infantile or more myopic initial mean refraction (Hirsch 1964, Gwiazda et al. 1993a, Howland et al. 1993, Zadnik and Mutti 1994, Drobe and Saint-André 1995); while emmetropization occurred during the pre-school years, nonetheless, it later showed a regression towards the initial infantile refractive state (Gwiazda et al. 1993a) (Figure 7-1)
- against-the-rule astigmatism (Hirsch 1964, Gwiazda et al. 1993a), but only in conjunction with infantile negative spherical equivalent refraction (Gwiazda et al. 1993a)
- less negative near point concave reading threshold (Drobe and Saint-André 1995)
- reduced accommodative amplitude and near point reading amplitude (Drobe and Saint-André 1995)

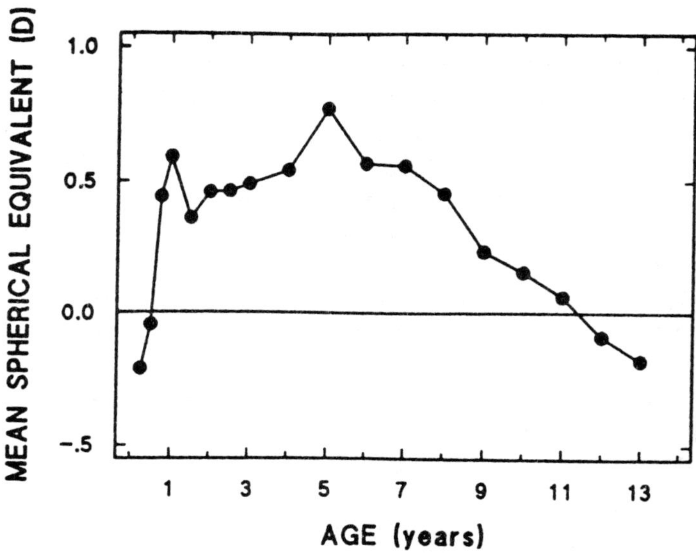

Figure 7-1 : Longitudinal manifest refractions (mean spherical equivalent) from 72 children fom birth to 13y (Reprinted with permission, Gwiazda et al. 1993a).

- reduced positive relative accommodation (Goss 1991b, Goss and Jackson 1996a), which was suggested to be secondary to the increased esophoria at near (Goss and Jackson 1996a)
- more positive near point binocular cross-cylinder (Goss 1991b, Drobe and Saint-André 1995)
- transient episode of pseudomyopia immediately prior to the onset of permanent myopia (Mei and Rong 1994)
- true or relative esophoria at near (Goss 1991b, Drobe and Saint-André 1995, Goss and Jackson 1996b), with a 1-3 prism diopter difference between refractive groups (Goss and Jackson 1996b)
- more convergent midpoint of the near fusional vergence range (Goss and Jackson 1996a)
- increased corneal power; however, the use of appropiate statistics to account for errors associated with multiple comparisons eliminated the initially significant group difference (Goss and Jackson 1995)
- increased ratio of axial length to corneal radius (AL/CR) (Grosvenor 1988, Goss and Jackson 1995); an AL/CR significantly greater than 3.0 is strongly suggestive of myopic development; while the AL/CR differed between refractive groups, the axial length, lens thickness and anterior chamber depth did not

TABLE 7-2: PREVALENCE OF MYOPIA IN OFFSPRING AS A FUNCTION OF PARENTAL HISTORY OF MYOPIA

INVESTIGATION	NEITHER PARENT MYOPIC (%)	ONE PARENT MYOPIC (%)	BOTH PARENTS MYOPIC (%)
Paul (1938)	10	30	60
Wold (1949)	35	49	
Keller (1973)	15	40	45
Ashton (1985)	11	16-25	33-46
Gwiazda et al. (1993a)	8	23	42
Yap et al. (1993)	7	26	45
Zadnik et al. (1994)	2-6	5-8	11-12
Goss & Jackson (1996c)	6	37	57

- a parental history of myopia (see Table 7-2); offsprings having 2 myopic parents demonstrated the greatest tendency towards myopia, those with no myopic parents showed the least, while those with one myopic parent exhibited intermediate values. In addition, Zadnik et al. (1994) indicated that in children with a parental history of myopia, the eyes were characterized by increased anterior and vitreous chamber depths and lower crystalline lens powers, while corneal powers were similar to those without a myopic parental history (Table 7-3).

POSSIBLE PREVENTIVE AND TREATMENT TECHNIQUES FOR MYOPIA

There are a variety of approaches and techniques that have been advocated over the years, primarily by optometrists, in an attempt to prevent, inhibit, and even reverse myopic presence especially in lower degrees of ametropia (Birnbaum 1994, Sherman and Press 1997). Although the intentions have been commendable, the results over the years have been mixed which, in part, have reflected our lack of understanding of some of the basic mechanisms. However, increased research in this area over the past two decades, which was instigated by the intriguing animal results of Torsten Wiesel, Josh Wallman, Tom Norton, Neville McBrien, Earl Smith and others, has provided important new insights (see Chapter 6).

Pharmacologic paralysis of accommodation. Especially with potent (and potentially dangerous) drugs such as atropine, most of the results involving paralysis of accommodation have demonstrated cessation of myopic progression. This is true for human (Gimbal 1973, Bedrossian 1979), as well as tree shrew and other lower species (McBrien et al. 1993). Over the years, it was believed that the basic mechanism involved the

TABLE 7-3: MEANS OF REFRACTIVE ERROR AND OCULAR COMPONENTS BY PARENTAL REFRACTIVE ERROR HISTORY CATEGORY WITH PREVALENT MYOPIC CHILDREN EXCLUDED (AT LEAST -0.75D OF MYOPIA IN EACH MERIDIAN), CONTROLLING FOR BOTH GRADE IN SCHOOL AND DIOPTER-HOURS (N=622 CHILDREN)*
(Zadnik et al. 1994)

MYOPIC PARENT CATEGORY	NO. OF CHILDREN	REFRACTIVE ERROR, D	CORNEAL POWER, D	LENS THICKNESS, mm	ANTERIOR CHAMBER DEPTH, mm	VITREOUS CHAMBER DEPTH, mm	CRYSTALLINE LENS POWER, D
BOTH	158	0.51	44.05	3.47	3.70	15.76	20.50
EITHER	290	0.62	43.91	3.48	3.66	15.71	20.66
NEITHER	214	0.72	44.03	3.49	3.62	15.57	20.85
P†	...	.01	.61	.56	.002	.01	.06

* Least-square means are estimated from analysis of covariance models.

† The significance probability is associated with the F test of the hypothesis of equality of the means.

biomechanical and IOP-related aspects of accommodation. Such explanations have never been wholly satisfactory. However, recent evidence in chicks has suggested a non-accommodative route (McBrien et al. 1993). This is believed to involve retinal neurotransmitters and related ocular growth hormones (McBrien et al. 1993, Goss and Wickham 1995), with the notion that such a mechanism is species-independent. This is a novel idea that deserves serious consideration and further testing, especially in certain children and young adults who are most susceptible to myopigenic factors. This idea is consistent with our conclusion that the biomechanical aspects of accommodation (and convergence) are insufficient to explain to any great extent myopic onset, development, and progression (see this chapter and Chapter 5).

Bifocals. Based on the above discussion, this may explain the mixed results of bifocal treatment for myopia in the general population of children. Several factors may account for this. First, based on our findings with respect to NITM, the near addition should probably equal the accommodative stimulus level to minimize blur-driven accommodation. Thus, for most children, a +3 diopter or even greater add would appear to be required for substantial effect. Other than to reestablish appropriate accommodation and vergence interactions at near, low-powered adds (i.e., +0.5D or so) may not be very beneficial to prevent myopic onset and progression. Second, the add should be worn during *all* near work activities, and this can be difficult to control in children. Third, the add should be fitted slightly higher than normal to force all near tasks to be performed through it and to prevent "peeking" above the near segment. And, fourth, bifocals may only be efficacious in specific subgroups of patients, such as those with near esophoria and demanding nearwork requirements (Figure 7-2). In addition, as suggested by Grosvenor (1989), instead of prescribing bifocals to individuals who are already myopic, it would be more beneficial to prescribe them prior to the onset of myopia in "at risk" individuals.

Vision therapy. Various forms of accommodative vision therapy have been advocated in the treatment of myopia (Avetisov 1989, Rosenblyum et al. 1989, Birnbaum 1993, Sherman and Press 1997), especially blur-based lens rock. For example, Avetisov (1989) found that the eventual frequency of myopia in an "at risk" group (i.e., having low accommodative reserves) who had received simple accommodative therapy was only 2.6% as compared with 31.1% in an untreated group. Clearly, such treatment would not be beneficial in already established myopia having an axial-length basis. However, such therapy might be beneficial in certain diagnostic subgroups. This might include cases of symptomatic NITM, patients who have the oculomotor potential and/or history of myopic progression, patients "at risk" of becoming myopic as a preventive measure (as the results of Avetisov

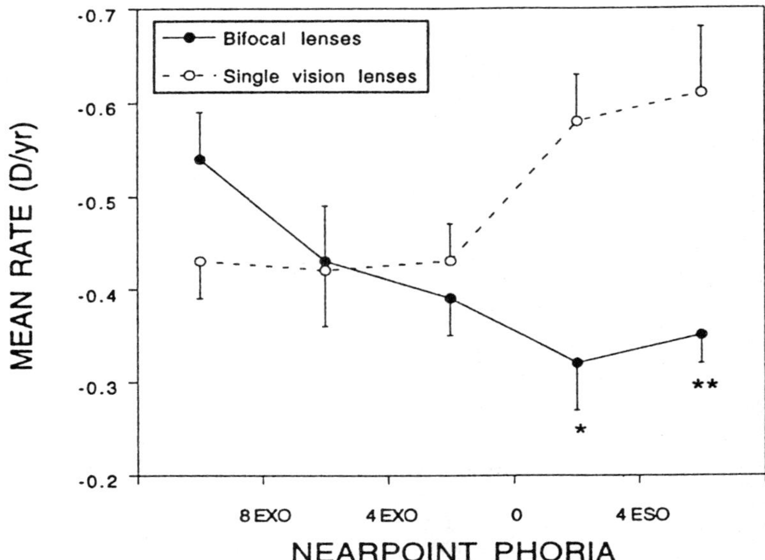

*Figure 7-2 : Mean rate of childhood myopic progression in diopters per year as a function of near point phoria and lens type. Asterisks indicate that the means for the bifocal lens wearers and the single vision lens wearers were significantly different (*P<0.001; **P<0.0005). The error bars are one standard error (Reprinted with permission, Goss and Uyesugi 1995).*

above suggest), the pre-myopic syndrome (Goss 1991b, Drobe and Saint-Andre 1995, Goss and Jackson 1996a) and the earliest stages of myopic development (Gwiazda 1995), and cases of frank pseudomyopia which may reflect a transitional phase towards permanent myopia (Mei and Rong 1994). Other related techniques might include distance visual imagery, relaxation procedures, and frequent rest periods during extended nearwork tasks. In addition, accommodative procedures under binocular viewing conditions (both congruent and non-congruent) should be helpful in developing normal accommodative and vergence interactions.

NOVEL DIAGNOSTIC AND THERAPEUTIC APPROACHES TO MYOPIA

A variety of novel approaches have evolved over the years in an attempt to understand the basic processes involved in myopigenesis, as well as to improve and expand upon conventional aspects related to myopia diagnosis and therapy. Some of these are briefly described below.

Surgery. The surgical approach to myopia has resulted in a wide array of techniques, with many being extreme in nature. For example, Russian ophthalmologists have injected liquid polymers with catalytic additives behind the globe into Tenon's capsule (Iomdina et al. 1989). This material then transforms into an elastic gel surrounding the posterior globe. Presence of this material stimulates collagen formation presumably by acting as a mechanical irritant, thus strengthening this most susceptible region of the sclera. This procedure has been used in some humans with very high and rapidly progressive myopia. In another technique used by both Russians and Americans in similar cases, grafting of donor posterior sclera onto a similar host region has been performed, again as a mechanical strengthening procedure (Nurmamedov et al. 1989). A less invasive treatment technique in vogue at present in the United States and many other countries of the world involves use of the excimer laser in patients having low to moderate degrees of myopia to mold the cornea surgically to compensate optically for the effectively over-powered eye (McDonnell 1995). While the technique now has FDA approval, careful psychophysical testing has yet to be done to determine any adverse effects on more subtle aspects of vision function, especially under relatively dim illumination in conjunction with glare sources as would be found during typical night-time driving conditions. Additional work is clearly needed here.

Auditory biofeedback. This can be a powerful conditioning tool to alter and/or optimize motor system responsivity (Ciuffreda and Goldrich 1983). Essentially, one hears a tone correlated with refractive state and attempts to use higher-level voluntary control and develop strategies to alter the tone in a specific way to affect accommodation in the desired manner. It has been demonstrated to be effective in shaping accommodative control in normals (Randle 1970, Cornsweet and Crane 1973). We have also successfully used it in our laboratory both in normals and in patients with various accommodative dysfunctions. If most lower degrees of myopia had a primary (accommodative) lenticular-basis, then auditory biofeedback could be a potent clinical tool in the reduction of myopia (Trachtman et al. 1981, Trachtman 1990). A commercial device has even been developed for such a purpose. Unfortunately, subsequent clinical testing by various investigators has shown it to be ineffective for general myopia reduction (Gallaway et al. 1987, Koslowe et al. 1991, Gilmartin et al. 1991, Angi et al. 1996), as most existing and in particular stable myopias have an axial-length basis. However, we have used our own laboratory system on selected patients, and have found it to be helpful in those with NITM/pseudomyopia (~1D or so) in which the accommodative mechanism is directly involved. Clearly, once axial-based myopia has developed, such training of the accommodative neurosensory and neuromuscular systems would not impact on this established component of the myopia. Improved accommodative ability, however, might prevent further development of myopia, especially in those individuals who perform considerable nearwork, have abnormal near accommodation, and/or have other risk factors for myopia. This area deserves further clinical consideration, especially in light of recent evidence suggesting a link between pseudomyopia of lenticular origin and permanent myopia of axial origin.

Biochemical analysis. However, perhaps the area we find most intriguing at the present time is the use of biochemical analysis to assist in the diagnosis and treatment of myopia, with its potential to predict refractive state, the timing of its development, and perhaps even its rate of progression. The recent convergence of key findings in human and animal studies (especially the tree shrew which is closely related to primates) makes such speculation even more exciting and inviting (see Goss and Wickham 1995, for an excellent review of this area). Again, the basic scientists dealing with their animal models of myopia must be given much of the credit. The biochemical aspects appear to provide the crucial link between accommodation/retinal defocus and myopic axial elongation. That is, *the accommodatively-related retinal defocus/image degradation appears to trigger specific biochemical changes in the sclera and related contiguous structures that results in posterior pole axial elongation.*

For example, glycosaminoglycans (GAGs) are involved in collagen fibrillogenesis (Avetisov et al. 1984, Balacco-Gabrieli 1989, Vinetskaya et al. 1989, Balacco-Gabrieli et al. 1993). GAGs influence collagen size and its organization, and they are highly represented in eye tissue. There has been increasing speculation that modification of collagen in the sclera of myopes occurs due to retinal defocus/image degradation effects, and that GAG metabolism might reflect this process (Goss and Wickham 1995). Uronic acids in the urine, which are related to and correlated with GAG metabolism, have been measured in human myopes and non-myopic controls (Balacco-Gabrieli et al. 1993). The uronic acid was 2-3 times greater in the myopes. Similarly, reduced levels of hydroxyproline (related to collagen accummulation) were found in both human blood serum levels (Vinetskaya et al. 1989) and human sclera (Avetisov et al. 1984), as well as tree shrew sclera (McBrien and Norton 1994, Norton and Rada 1995). Thus, in addition to providing increased evidence for the tree shrew as a reasonable model for human myopia, the results suggested that myopic axial elongation was the result not only of simple biomechanical scleral stretching but also to changes in its biochemical constitution (Guggenheim and McBrien 1996).

While the use of biochemical probes is highly speculative in nature and only in its infancy, one can begin to conjure up images of the optometrist collecting urine, blood, and perhaps even minute tissue samples from the anterior sclera of one's patients to perform such biochemical analyses, especially in children and young adults "at risk" of becoming myopic. Such additional physiologically-based information could be of use in the prevention and early intervention of myopia. Clearly, further developments at both the basic and clinical levels are needed to assess the viability of such biochemical analyses in the clinical management of myopia.

SUMMARY

During this century, a considerable body of information has amassed that may be relevant to the topic of accommodation, nearwork and myopia. Clearly, there are still many unresolved questions and much for future researchers to study as we approach the next century and millenium. Thus, it appears to be most appropriate at this time to sort through this information, take with us that which seems reasonable and holds up to scientific scrutiny, and, lastly, to provide a vision for future directions of basic research, clinical investigation, and clinical patient care.

REFERENCES

Abdalla MI, Hamdi M. Applanation ocular tension in myopia and emmetropia. Br J Ophthalmol. 1970; 54: 122-5.

Adams AJ. Axial length elongation, not corneal curvature, as a basis of adult-onset myopia. Am J Optom Physiol Opt. 1987; 64: 150-2.

Adams DW, McBrien NA. A longitudinal study of adult-onset myopia and adult progression of myopia- two year refractive error and axial dimension results. Invest Ophthalmol Vis Sci (Suppl). 1992; 33: 712.

Angi MR, Caucci S, Pilotto E, Racano E, Rupolo G, Sabbadin E. Changes in myopia, visual acuity, and psychological distress after biofeedback visual training. Optom Vis Sci. 1996; 73: 35-42.

Ashton GC. Segregation analysis of ocular refraction and myopia. Human Heredity. 1985; 35: 232-9.

Avetisov ES. A three-factor theory of myopia- prevention and progression checking. Proceedings of the International Symposium, Myopia: Pathogenesis, Prevention, Progression, and Complications. Helmholtz Research Institute of Eye Disease, Moscow; 1989: 9-15.

Avetisov ES, Savitskaya NF, Vinetskaya MI, Iomdina EN. A study of biochemical and biomechanical qualities of normal and myopic eye sclera in humans of different age groups. Metab Ped Systemic Ophthalmol. 1984; 7: 183-8.

Balacco-Gabrieli C. Aetiopathogenesis of degenerative myopia: a hypothesis. Proceedings of the International Symposium, Myopia: Pathogenesis, Prevention, Progression, and Complications. Helmholtz Research Institute of Eye Disease, Moscow; 1989: 15-8.

Balacco-Gabrieli C, Moramarco A, Kozich W, Feher J, Filipec M, Hoskovcova H, Pezzulli S. Preliminary study of glycosaminoglycan metabolism in high myopia. Ital J Ophthalmol. 1993; 7: 87-9.

Baldwin WR. Corneal curvature changes in high myopia versus corneal curvature changes in low myopia. Am J Optom Arch Am Acad Optom. 1962; 39: 349-55.

Baldwin WR. The relationship between axial length of the eye and certain other anthropometric measurements of myopes. Am J Optom Arch Am Acad Optom. 1964; 41: 513-22.

Baldwin WR. Some relationships between ocular, anthropometric and refractive variables in myopia. PhD thesis. Bloomington: University of Indiana School of Optometry; 1965.

Barraquer J. Coloquio sobre miopia; 1974. Cited in Kelly TSB. In: Fledelius HC, Alsbirk PH, Goldschmidt E, eds. Third International Conference on Myopia, Copenhagen. The Hague: Dr W. Junk Publishers. Doc Ophthal Proc Series. 1981; 23: 109-16.

Bedrossian RH. The effect of atropine on myopia. Am J Ophthalmol. 1979; 86: 713-7.

Birnbaum MH. Optometric Management of Nearpoint Vision Disorders. Boston: Butterworth-Heinemann; 1993: 303-9.

Bullimore MA, Gilmartin B, Royston JM. Steady-state accommodation and ocular biometry in late-onset myopia. Doc Ophthalmol. 1992; 80: 143-55.

Castrén JA, Pohjola S. Refraction and scleral rigidity. Acta Ophthalmol. 1961; 39: 1011-4.

Cheng HM, Omah SS, Kwong KK, Xiong J, Woods BT, Brady TJ. Shape of the myopic eye as seen with high-resolution magnetic resonance imaging. Optom Vis Sci. 1992; 69: 698-701.

Ciuffreda KJ, Colburn C, Wallis D. Effect of stimulus duration and dioptric demand on transient myopia. Invest Ophthalmol Vis Sci (Suppl). 1996; 37: S164.

Ciuffreda KJ, Goldrich SG. Oculomotor biofeedback therapy. Internat Rehab Med. 1983; 5: 111-7.

Ciuffreda KJ, Ordoñez X. Abnormal transient myopia in symptomatic individuals after sustained nearwork. Optom Vis Sci. 1995; 72: 506-10.

Coleman DJ. Unified model for the accommodative mechanism. Am J Ophthalmol. 1970; 69: 1063-79.

Cornsweet TN, Crane HD. Training the visual accommodation system. Vis Res. 1973; 13: 713-5.

Curtin BJ. The Myopias: Basic Science and Clinical Management. Philadelphia: Harper & Row; 1985.

Curtin BJ, Iwamoto T, Renaldo DP. Normal and staphylomatous sclera of high myopia—an electron microscopic study. Arch Ophthalmol. 1979; 97: 912-5.

Curtin BJ, Teng CC. Scleral changes in pathological myopia. Trans Am Acad Ophthalmol Otolaryngol. 1958; 62: 777-88.

David R, Zangwill LM, Tessler Z, Yassur Y. The correlation between intraocular pressure and refractive status. Arch Ophthalmol. 1985; 103: 1812-5.

Donders FC. On the Anomalies of Accommodation and Refraction of the Eye. trans. Moore WD. London: The New Sydenham Society; 1864.

Drance SM. The significance of the diurnal tension variations in normal and glaucomatous eyes. Arch Ophthalmol. 1960; 64: 494-501.

Drobe B, Saint-André R. The pre-myopic syndrome. Ophthal Physiol Opt. 1995; 15: 375-8.

Duke-Elder S. The phasic variations in the ocular tension in primary glaucoma. Am J Ophthalmol. 1952; 35: 1-21.

Edwards MH, Brown B. Intraocular pressure in a selected sample of myopic and non-myopic Chinese children. Optom Vis Sci. 1993; 70: 15-7.

Edwards MH, Brown B. IOP in myopic children: the relationship between increases in IOP and the development of myopia. Ophthal Physiol Opt. 1996; 243-6.

Ehrlich DL. Near vision stress: vergence adaptation and accommodative fatigue. Ophthal Physiol Opt. 1987; 7: 353-7.

Erickson P. Mathematical model for predicting dioptric effects of optical parameter changes in the eye. Am J Optom Physiol Opt. 1977; 54: 226-33.

Fisher RF. Is the vitreous necessary for accommodation in man? Brit J Ophthalmol. 1983; 67: 206.

Fledelius HC. Refractive components in aniso- and isometropia. In: Fledelius HC, Alsbirk PH, Goldschmidt E, eds. Third International Conference on Myopia, Copenhagen. The Hague: Dr W. Junk Publishers. Doc Ophthal Proc Series. 1981; 28: 89-95.

Fledelius HC. Adult onset myopia— oculometric features. Acta Ophthalmol Scand. 1995; 73: 397-401.

Franceschetti A, Gernet H. Importance of ultrasonic echography for measurements of the optical components of the eye. Trans Am Acad Ophthalmol Otol. 1965a; 69: 465-73.

Franceschetti A, Gernet H. Uber optische Groben bei leichter und hoher myopie auf grund echographischer befunde, Graefe's Arch Ophthalmol. 1965b; 168: 1-16. Cited in: Gernet H. Oculometric findings in myopia. In: Fledelius HC, Alsbirk PH, Goldschmidt E, eds. Third International Conference on Myopia, Copenhagen. The Hague: Dr W. Junk Publishers. Doc Ophthalmol Proc Series. 1981: 28: 71-7.

Franceschetti A, Luyckx J. Study of the emmetropization effect of the crystalline lens by ultrasonic echography. Am J Ophthalmol. 1966; 61: 1096-100.

Francois J, Goes F. Comparative study of ultrasonic biometry of emmetropes and myopes with special regard to the heredity of myopia. In: Gitter KA, Keeney AH, Sarin LK, Meyer D, eds. Ophthalmic Ultrasound-proceedings of the 4th international congress of ultrasonography in ophthalmology, Philadelphia. St. Louis: C.V. Mosby Co.; 1969: 165-80.

Gallaway M, Pearl SM, Winkelstein AM, Scheiman M. Biofeedback training of visual acuity and myopia: a pilot study. Am J Optom Physiol Opt. 1987, 64: 62-71.

Garner LF, Chung KM, Grosvenor TP, Mohidin N. Ocular dimensions and refractive power in Malay and Melanesian children. Ophthal Physiol Opt. 1990; 10:234-8.

Garner LF, Yap M, Scott R. Crystalline lens power in myopia. Optom Vis Sci. 1992; 69: 863-5.

Gernet H. Oculometric findings in myopia. In: Fledelius HC, Alsbirk PH, Goldschmidt E, eds. Third International Conference on Myopia, Copenhagen. The Hague: Dr W. Junk Publishers. Doc Ophthal Proc Series. 1981; 28: 71-7.

Gilmartin B, Gray LS, Winn B. The amelioration of myopia using biofeedback of accommodation: a review. Ophthal Physiol Opt. 1991; 11: 304-13.

Gimbel HV. The control of myopia with atropine. Can J Ophthalmol. 1973; 8: 527-32.

Goss DA. Childhood myopia. In: Grosvenor T, Flom MC, eds. Refractive Anomalies-Research and Clinical Applications. Boston: Butterworth-Heinemann; 1991a: 81-103.

Goss DA. Clinical accommodation and heterophoria findings preceding juvenile onset of myopia. Optom Vis Sci. 1991b; 68: 110-6.

Goss DA, Erickson P. Meridional corneal components of myopia progression in young adults and children. Am J Optom Physiol Opt. 1987; 64: 475-81.

Goss DA, Erickson P, Cox VD. Prevalence and pattern of adult myopia progression in a general optometric practice population. Am J Optom Physiol Opt. 1985; 62: 470-7.

Goss DA, Jackson TW. Ocular dioptric components prior to youth onset of myopia. Optom Vis Sci (Suppl). 1992; 69: 110.

Goss DA, Jackson TW. Clinical findings before the onset of myopia in youth. I. Ocular optical components. Optom Vis Sci. 1995; 72: 870-8.

Goss DA, Jackson TW. Clinical findings before the onset of myopia in youth: 2. Zone of clear single binocular vision. Optom Vis Sci. 1996a; 73: 263-68.

Goss DA, Jackson TW. Clinical findings before the onset of myopia in youth: 3. Heterophoria. Optom Vis Sci. 1996b; 73: 269-78.

Goss DA, Jackson TW. Clinical findings before the onset of myopia in youth: 4. Parental history of myopia. Optom Vis Sci. 1996c; 73: 279-82.

Goss DA, Uyesugi EF. Effectiveness of bifocal control of childhood myopia progression as a function of near point phoria and binocular cross-cylinder. J Optom Vis Dev. 1995; 26: 11-7.

Goss DA, Wickham MG. Retinal-image mediated ocular growth as a mechanism for juvenile onset myopia and for emmetropization. Doc Ophthalmol. 1995; 90: 341-75.

Greene PR. Mechanical considerations in myopia. In: Grosvenor T, Flom MC, eds. Refractive Anomalies— Research and Clinical Applications; 1991: 287-300.
Grosvenor T. High axial length/corneal radius ratio as a risk factor in the development of myopia. Am J Optom Physiol Opt. 1988; 65: 689-96.
Grosvenor T. Myopia: what can we do about it clinically? Optom Vis Sci. 1989; 66: 415-9.
Grosvenor T. Refractive component changes in adult-onset myopia: evidence from five studies. Clin Exp Optom. 1994; 77: 196-205.
Grosvenor T, Scott R. Comparison of refracting components in youth-onset and early adult-onset myopia. Optom Vis Sci. 1991; 68: 204-9.
Grosvenor T, Scott R. Three-year changes in refraction and its components in youth-onset and early adult-onset myopia. Optom Vis Sci. 1993; 70: 677-83.
Grosvenor T, Scott R. Role of the axial length/corneal radius ratio in determining the refractive state of the eye. Optom Vis Sci. 1994; 71: 573-9.
Guggenheim JA, McBrien NA. Form-deprivation myopia induces activation of scleral matrix metalloproteinase-2 in tree shrew. Invest Ophthalmol Vis Sci. 1996; 37: 1380-95.
Gwiazda J, Bauer J, Thorn F, Held R. A dynamic relationship between myopia and blur-driven accommodation in school-aged children. Vis Res. 1995; 35: 1299-304.
Gwiazda J, Thorn F, Bauer J, Held R. Emmetropization and the progression of manifest refraction in children followed from infancy to puberty. Clin Vis Sci. 1993a; 8: 337-44.
Gwiazda J, Thorn F, Bauer J, Held R. Myopic children show insufficient accommodative response to blur. Invest Ophthalmol Vis Sci. 1993b; 34: 690-4.
Harrie RP. Factors in emmetropization. In: Ossoinig KC, ed. Ophthalmic Echography. Proceedings of the 10th SIDUO Congress 1984. Dordrecht: Martinus Nijhoff/Dr W. Junk Publishers; 1987: 65-72.
Held R, Gwiazda JE, Thorn F, Bauer JA. Changes in accommodative responsiveness are linked to the development of myopia in children. Invest Ophthal Vis Sci (Supp.). 1994;35:1735.
Hirsch MJ. Predictability of refraction at age 14 on the basis of testing at age 6-interim report from the Ojai longitudinal study of refraction. Am J Optom Arch Am Acad Optom. 1964; 41: 567-73.
Howland HC, Waite S, Peck L. Early focusing history predicts later refractive state: a longitudinal photorefractive study. In: Noninvasive Assessment of the Visual System Technical Digest 1993. Washington, DC: Optical Society of America. 1993; 3: 210-3.
Hung LF, Smith EL III. Extended-wear, soft, contact lenses produce hyperopia in young monkeys. Optom Vis Sci. 1996; 73: 579-84.
Iomdina EN, Vinetskaya MI, Andreyeva LD. The experimental basis for using a non-surgical method to strengthen the sclera in progressive myopia. Proceedings of the International Symposium, Myopia: Pathogenesis, Prevention, Progression, and Complications. Helmholtz Research Institute of Eye Disease, Moscow; 1989: 180-3.
Javitt JC, Chiang YP. The socioeconomic aspects of laser refractive surgery. Arch Ophthalmol. 1994; 112: 1526-30.
Jiang BC, Woessner WM. Vitreous chamber elongation is responsible for myopia development in a young adult. Optom Vis Sci. 1996; 73: 231-4.
Keller JT. A comparison of the refractive status of myopic children and their parents. Am J Optom Arch Am Acad Optom. 1973; 50: 206-11.
Kent R. Acquired myopia of prematurity. Am J Optom Arch Am Acad Optom. 1963; 40: 247-56.
Koslowe KC, Spierer A, Rosner M, Belkin M. Evaluation of Accommotrac biofeedback training for myopia control. Optom Vis Sci. 1991; 68: 338-43.
Lancaster WZ, Williams ER. New light on the theory of accommodation with practical applications. Trans Am Acad Ophthalmol Otolaryngol. 1914; 19: 170-95.

Larsen JS. The sagittal growth of the eye, part I: Measurement of the depth of the anterior segment from birth to puberty. Acta Ophthalmol. 1971a; 49: 239-62.

Larsen JS. The sagittal growth of the eye, part II: Ultrasonic measurement of the axial diameter of the lens and anterior segment from birth to puberty. Acta Ophthalmol. 1971b; 49: 427-40.

Liu KR, Chen MS, Ko LS. Electron microscopic studies of the scleral collagen fiber in excessively high myopia. J Formosan Med Assoc. 1986; 85: 1032-8.

Mawas J. Introduction a l'etude de la myopie et des chorioretinites myopiques. Bull Soc d'Opht de Paris 1934; 1: 549-601. Cited in Friedman B. Stress upon the ocular coats: Effects of scleral curvature, scleral thickness, and intra-ocular pressure. The Eye, Ear, Nose and Throat Monthly. 1966; 45: 59-66.

McBrien NA, Millodot M. A biometric investigation of late-onset myopic eyes. Acta Ophthalmol. 1987; 65: 461-8.

McBrien NA, Moghaddam HO, Reeder AP. Atropine reduces experimental myopia and eye enlargement via a nonaccommodative mechanism. Invest Ophthalmol Vis Sci. 1993; 34: 205-15.

McBrien NA, Norton TT. Prevention of collagen crosslinking increases form deprivation myopia in tree shrew. Exp Eye Res. 1994; 59: 475-86.

McDonnell PJ. Excimer laser corneal surgery: new strategies and old enemies. Invest Ophthalmol Vis Sci. 1995; 36: 4-8.

Mei Q, Rong Z. Early signs of myopia in Chinese schoolchildren. Optom Vis Sci. 1994; 71: 14-6.

Norton TT, Rada JA. Reduced extracellular matrix in mammalian sclera with induced myopia. Vis Res. 1995; 35: 1271-81.

Nurmamedov NN, Atameredova GH, Toydzhanova GH. A one-graft alloscleroplasty in progressive myopia. Proceedings of the International Symposium, Myopia: Pathogenesis, Prevention, Progression, and Complications. Helmholtz Research Institute of Eye Disease, Moscow; 1989: 157-60.

Ong E. Oculomotor interactions and nearwork-induced transient myopia in late-onset myopes. PhD thesis. SUNY/State College of Optometry, New York City; 1996.

Ong E, Ciuffreda KJ. Nearwork-induced transient myopia- a critical review. Doc Ophthalmol. 1995; 91: 57-85.

Otsuka J, Sugata T, Araki M. The aetiology of myopia as considered from the differences in the refractive components of the right and left eyes. In: Fledelius HC, Alsbirk PH, Goldschmidt E, eds. Third International Conference on Myopia, Copenhagen. The Hague: Dr W. Junk Publishers. Doc Ophthal Proc Series. 1981; 28: 79-87.

Parssinen O, Lyyra AL. Myopia and myopic progression among schoolchildren: a three-year follow-up study. Invest Ophthalmol Vis Sci. 1993; 34: 2794-802.

Paul L. Untersuchungen über der erbliche Entstehung der Kurzsichtigkeit. I. Mitteilung. Von Graefes Arch Ophthalmol. 1938; 139: 378-402. Cited in: Goss DA, Jackson TW. Clinical findings before the onset of myopia in youth: 4. Parental history of myopia. Optom Vis Sci. 1996c; 73: 279-82.

Perkins ES. Ocular volume and ocular rigidity. Exp Eye Res. 1981b; 33: 141-5.

Phelps CD, Woolson RF, Kolker AE, Becker B. Diurnal variation in intraocular pressure. Am J Ophthalmol. 1974; 77: 367-7.

Phillips JR, McBrien NA. Form deprivation myopia: elastic properties of sclera. Ophthal Physiol Opt. 1995; 15: 357-62.

Pruett RC. Progressive myopia and intraocular pressure: what is the linkage? a literature review. Acta Ophthalmol (Suppl). 1988; 185: 117-27.

Randle RJ. Volitional control of visual accommodation. AGARD Conf Proc. 1970; 82: 715-7.

Rosenblyum YZ, Matz KA, Lokhtina NN, Stishkovskaya GA, Medvetskaya GA. Functional methods to prevent myopia and its progression. Proceedings of the International Symposium, Myopia: Pathogenesis, Prevention, Progression, and Complications. Helmholtz Research Institute of Eye Disease, Moscow; 1989: 70-5.

Rosenfield M. Accommodation and myopia: are they related? J Behav Optom. 1994; 5: 3-11.

Rosenfield M, Ciuffreda KJ, Hung GK, Gilmartin B. Tonic accommodation: a review. I. Basic aspects. Ophthal Physiol Opt. 1993; 13: 266-84.

Rosenfield M, Ciuffreda KJ, Hung GK, Gilmartin B. Tonic accommodation: a review. II. Adaptation and clinical implications. Ophthal Physiol Opt. 1994; 14: 265-77.

Rosenfield M, Ciuffreda KJ, Novogrodsky L. Contribution of accommodation and disparity vergence to transient nearwork-induced myopic shifts. Ophthal Physiol Opt. 1992a; 12: 433-6.

Rosenfield M, Ciuffreda KJ, Novogrodsky L, Yu A, Gillard M. Sustained near-vision does indeed induce myopia! Invest Ophthalmol Vis Sci (Suppl). 1992b; 33: 710.

Sato T. The causes and prevention of acquired myopia. Yokohama: Helarudo Printing Co. Ltd.; 1957.

Scott R, Grosvenor T. Structural model for emmetropic and myopic eyes. Ophthal Physiol Opt. 1993; 13: 41-7.

Sherman A, Press LJ. Myopia control therapy. In: Press LJ, ed. Applied Concepts in Vision Therapy. St. Louis: Mosby; 1997: 298-309.

Smith EL III, Hung LF, Harwerth RS. Effects of optically-induced blur on the refractive status of young monkeys. Vis Res. 1994; 34: 293-301.

Sorsby A. Biology of the eye as an optical system. In: Tasman W, ed. Duane's Clinical Ophthalmology, vol. 1. Philadelphia: J. B. Lippincott Co.; 1994: (34) 1-17.

Sorsby A, Benjamin B, Davey JB, Sheridan M, Tanner JM. Emmetropia and its aberrations, a study in the correlation of the optical components of the eye. Med Res Council Special Report Series No. 293. London: Her Majesty's Stationery Office; 1957.

Sorsby A, Leary GA. A longitudinal study of refraction and its components during growth. Med Res Council Special Report Series no. 309. London: Her Majesty's Stationery Office; 1970.

Sorsby A, Leary GA, Richards MJ. Correlation ametropia and component ametropia. Vis Res. 1962; 2: 309-13.

Stenström S. Untersuchungen über die variation und kovariation der optischen elemente des menschlichen auges. Acta Ophthalmologica (Suppl). 1946; 26. Cited in Sorsby A. Biology of the eye as an optical system. In: Tasman W, ed. Duane's Clinical Ophthalmology, vol. 1. Philadelphia: J. B. Lippincott Co.; 1994: (34) 1-17.

Stenström S. Variations and correlations of the optical components of the eye. In: Sorsby A, ed. Modern Trends in Ophthalmology, vol. 2, 2nd ed. New York: Paul B. Hoeber, Inc.; 1947: 87-102.

Stenström S. Investigation of the variation and the correlation of the optical elements of human eyes, trans. Woolf D. Am J Optom Arch Am Acad Optom. 1948; 25: 218-32, 286-99, 340-50, 388-97, 438-49, 496-504.

Stoddard KB. Physiological limitations on the function, production and elimination of ametropia. Am J Optom Arch Am Acad Optom. 1942; 19: 112-8.

Storey JK, Tromans C, Rabie E. Continuous biometry of the crystalline lens during accommodation. In: Sampaolesi R, ed. Ultrasonography in Ophthalmology. Dordrecht: Kluwer Academic Publishers; 1990: 117-23.

Tokoro T, Kabe S. Relation between changes in the ocular refraction and refractive components and development of the myopia. Acta Societatis Ophthalmologicae Japonicae 1964; 68: 1240-53. Cited in Goss DA. Childhood myopia. In: Grosvenor T, Flom

MC, eds. Refractive Anomalies-Research and Clinical Applications. Boston: Butterworth-Heinemann; 1991: 81-103.

Tomlinson A, Phillips CI. Applanation tension and axial length of the eyeball. Br J Ophthalmol. 1970; 54: 548-53.

Tomlinson A, Phillips CI. Unequal axial length of eyeball and ocular tension. Acta Ophthalmol. 1972; 50: 872-6.

Trachtman JN. The Etiology of Visual Disorders- a Neuroscience Model. Santa Ana, CA: Optom Ext Prog Foundation; 1990.

Trachtman JN, Giambalvo V, Feldman J. Biofeedback of accommodation to reduce functional myopia. Biofeed Self-Regulation. 1981; 6: 547-64.

Tron EJ. Variationsstatistische Untersuchungen u. Refraktion. Graefes Arch Ophthal; 1929: 122: 1. Cited in Sorsby A, Benjamin B, Davey JB, Sheridan M, Tanner JM. Emmetropia and its aberrations, a study in the correlation of the optical components of the eye. Med Res Council Special Report Series No. 293. London: Her Majesty's Stationery Office; 1957.

Tron EJ. The optical elements of the refractive power of the eye. In: Ridley F, Sorsby A, eds. Modern Trends in Ophthahlmol, vol. 1. New York: Paul B. Hoeber; 1940: 245-55.

Van Alphen GWHM. On emmetropia and ametropia. Ophthalmol (Suppl). 1961; 142: 1-92.

Vinetskaya MI, Boltaeva ZK, Iomdina EN. Some metabolic features of connective tissue in progressive myopia. Proceedings of the International Symposium, Myopia: Pathogenesis, Prevention, Progression, and Complications. Helmholtz Research Institute of Eye Disease, Moscow; 1989: 58-61.

Wold KC. Hereditary myopia. Arch Ophthalmol. 1949; 42: 225-37.

Yap M, Wu M, Liu M, Lee FL, Wang SH. Role of heredity in the genesis of myopia. Ophthal Physiol Opt. 1993; 13: 316-9.

Zadnik K, Mutti DO. Can we foretell childhood myopia? Rev Optom. 1994; 131: 43-4.

Zadnik K, Satariano WA, Mutti DO, Sholtz RI, Adams AJ. The effect of parental history of myopia on children's eye size. J Am Med Assoc. 1994; 271: 1323-7.

Index

Compiled by Jane Paula Plass, O.D.

NOTES

NOTES

NOTES